This book is for you

- f   depleted

- feel more in tune with your body

- support the reversal of a chronic health condition

- naturally choose food and exercise that support your well-being

- appreciate your body's innate healing wisdom

- drop and release some weight effortlessly and permanently

- be reminded and inspired to live a life that FEELS good

- slow the decline! And be able to say "Yes! The best is yet to come!"

Reading *Eat Dance Shine* may change your life ... and enable you to push back the years, by guiding you on the best ways to nourish your body and mind so that you can flourish.

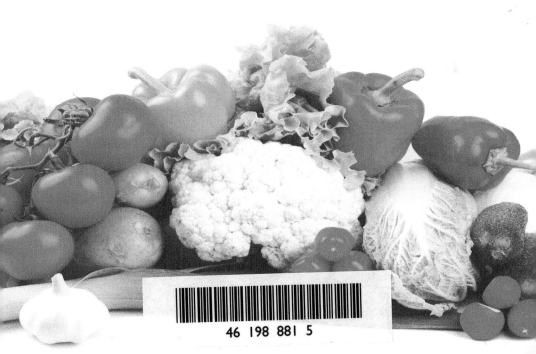

What people are saying about Michele

Jason Vale, aka 'Juice Master' bestselling author of twelve books on health, addiction and juicing

"*Eat Dance Shine* – follow its recommendations and you will notice increased vitality and longevity."

Debbie Rosas, Founder and CEO Nia Technique

"Paying attention to what we put into our body, mind, emotions, and spirit is key to staying healthy, well, and happy. Michele's wisdom provides inspiration and motivation to do just that, giving us all tools we can use to look good, feel good, and thrive in our body."

Marilyn Whyman, student

"I absolutely love my Nia classes. Michele is an amazing and gifted teacher. From the minute I walk into her class, I feel myself relax and really look forward to the next hour. I am never disappointed. Her classes are not only fun, but her routines energise me. I feel a different person when I leave. I believe Nia awakens the mind, spirit and body."

Julia, student

"For me, aged 69, Nia is the most uplifting form of exercise I've come across, and I've tried lots! Nia is so enjoyable to do – you can do it at any age as it's done at different levels within the class. I have problems with my knees and also occasional back pain. After only three classes, I can already feel the improvement in my body. Nia is gentle yet energising at the same time, and I particularly love dancing to the different music rhythms."

Debbie Harrington, student

"Makes me feel like I have moved and unlocked some stiff areas in my body; lovely people, lovely teacher."

Christine Orzel, student

"Nia is everything medicinal without the side effects. Nia is very clever; it has this slow release valve that keeps me well in-between classes."

Ann Bastow, student

"I attended Michele's Saturday morning Nia class. The addition of two drummers, who also sang, lifted everyone's mood and I personally found myself high on energy during and after the session. A great workout. Loved it!"

Joy Simmons, student

"A huge inspiration; it was even better than I imagined it was going to be. It was so positive and joyful, one cannot help but want to weave it into one's life!"

Sue, student

"Nia is simply a place for me, where I am not wife nor mother, not daughter nor sister."

Mariana Ingleby, student

"Simple things like getting up unaided, bending down to pick up a rubber band, or filling up the salt container of my dishwasher without doing my back in, would not be possible for me without Nia. Apart from being a lot of fun with great music, now in my seventies, Nia is an absolute must! Thank you, Michele."

Ann Worrall, student

"Over the years, Michele has taught me to be gentle with myself, to listen to my body, and to look for the pleasure. She uses few words, but those she does takes me into an imagination of movement rather than a physical description. Michele has a lightness of touch, a ready smile and a 'yes, we can' attitude. I love it!"

Michele Kaye MSc
Nutrition, Black Belt Nia teacher

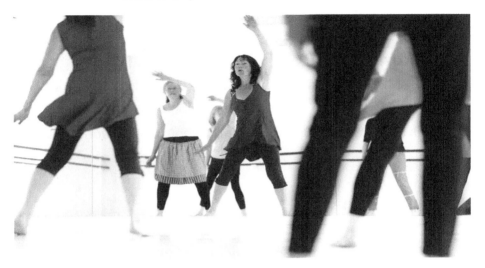

All my life, I have been passionate about the human body and how it creates health. This is what led me to become a biology teacher. My love of nature and all things natural goes back to early childhood, walking with my father in woods and gardens, appreciating all of life with curiosity and reverence. I am happy to say I grew up with cats and a dog as well as being a fanatically horsey teenager. My idea of heaven was spending the whole day at the stables, mucking out horses, riding, and generally helping out at the riding school. As an older teenager, the horse scene lost its appeal, and while my love for horses, and all animals, never faded, my passion for dancing replaced the riding. Several times a week, during my sixth form A level years, I would go to Manchester University discos, not to socialise but to dance.

After my A levels, I studied physiology with biochemistry (BSc) at Leeds University followed by medical research at Oxford University, then nutrition (MSc) and a Postgraduate Certificate in Education (PGCE), both at the University of London. Teaching came next, and over a 15-year period I taught mainly biology and health education, with some general science, mathematics and chemistry at secondary school level.

Marrying and having three children, Joseph, Leo and Flora, gave me a wonderful and enriching opportunity to put into practice all the nutrition I had learned academically as well as via avid reading and researching, including the importance of breastfeeding and delaying introducing wheat and dairy.

Further study of reiki and Emotional Freedom Technique (EFT), as well as a Raw Nutritional Science diploma, expanded my knowledge into the holistic arena, and I began my private practice about 15 years ago as a Healthy Living Coach, seeing clients individually, leading talks and holding Green Nutrition Workshops.

My love of dancing and moving expressively to music, eventually led me, in my late forties, to train as a Nia teacher. Nia, a holistic movement practice that originated from California, was started in the early 1980s . I have been teaching Nia since 2007, and during an eight-year period I completed several trainings, culminating in the Nia Black Belt in 2014.

My background as a biology teacher, nutritionist, Healthy Living Coach and EFT practitioner combine wonderfully with the holistically healing principles of Nia. During these last eight years, I have been teaching four to five classes of Nia each week, being inspired to keep supple, fit and happy while teaching women of all ages, shapes and sizes, who are also committed to their well-being. I see myself dancing and juicing well into my nineties and intend to bring many students, clients, family and friends along with me!

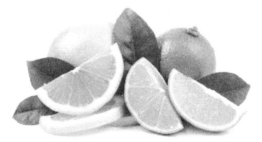

"It's always a good time to begin."

Unknown

*"My mission in life is
not merely to survive,
but to thrive."*

Maya Angelou

*"What you learn is that each decade
brings a new set of possibilities.
I have never felt more confident in myself,
more clear on who I am as a woman.
But I am constantly thinking about my own
health and making sure I'm
eating right and getting exercise
and watching the aches and pains.
I want to be this really fly
[awesome] 80-90 year old"*

First Lady Michelle Obama

Why feel your age when you could feel amazing!

EAT DANCE SHINE

How to come alive, gain energy and push back the years

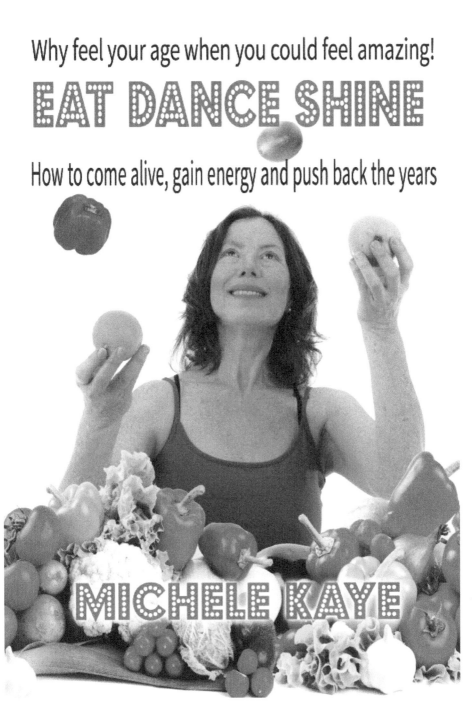

MICHELE KAYE

Foreword by Debbie Rosas
Founder of The Nia Technique

Published by
Filament Publishing Ltd
16 Croydon Road, Waddon, Croydon,
Surrey, CR0 4PA, United Kingdom.
+44(0)20 8688 2598
www.filamentpublishing.com

© Michele Kaye 2016

ISBN 978-1-910819-66-1

The right of Michele Kaye to be identified as the author of
this work has been asserted by her in accordance with the
Designs and Copyright Act 1988.

Printed by IngramSpark

Cartoons by Sarah Boyce   boycedavies@yahoo.com

This book is not intended as a substitute for the medical advice of
physicians. The reader should regularly consult a physician in matters
relating to his/her health and particularly with respect to any symptoms
that may require diagnosis or medical attention.

Table of Contents

List of Recipes

Acknowledgements

Writing a book cannot be done alone. There are many people I would like to thank for assisting me.

Firstly, my father for being an inspiring bookseller and writer, and my mother for leading the way, by writing two books of her own, in her early nineties.

Janey Lee Grace's coaching was invaluable, without which I would never have put pen to paper. She always believed in me, saying things like, "Wow, you really have got a book in you!"

I thank Chris Day of Filament Publishing for his genuine passion and enthusiasm for getting a book out into the world and his incredible patience. Flat out busy, Chris always had time to discuss a small detail that was important to me, as positive and encouraging as anyone would dream their publisher to be.

A big thank you to cartoonist extraordinaire and friend, Sarah Boyce (http://www.boycecartoons.wordpress.com/) whose cartoons make me laugh out loud. Her humour brightens up each chapter.

I am deeply grateful to Debbie Rosas and Carlos AyaRosas, co-creators of Nia, and to Ann Christiansen, Nia trainer, for the movement and lifestyle practice, Nia, which has changed my body and my life. Way beyond fitness, Nia teaches me to take mindfulness off the dance floor and into my daily life.

I thank my students and clients. It is wonderful to share Nia and nutrition with you and watch you grow.

Dear lifelong friends, Bea, Dawn, Pauline, Ann and Tamara, thank you for the countless hours and years discussing and debating our passion for natural health and nutrition. Many other dear friends too, who gave me all the encouragement that I needed, and listened patiently to a writer's woes.

I thank my family who sampled weird and wonderful juices, salads and stews over the years. My dear husband who ongoingly stands by me, patiently listening to many hours of nutritional "Did you know … ?" questions. On many occasions, he would enter the kitchen, only to find me jazz dancing around, or throwing funky tae kwon do punches and kicks, in time to some great Nia music. I appreciate all the creative ideas offered by my grown-up children, Joseph, Leo and Flora, as well as their wonderfully honest feedback (that can only come from your own kids!).

Finally, I thank the plant kingdom and the elements, seen and unseen, for without them, we would have no food.

Foreword by Debbie Rosas
Founder of The Nia Technique

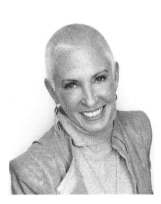

I have spent most of my life researching how to live and move in my body in healthy and meaningful ways. What started out as a personal journey has developed into a business, the business of the body. I believe everybody is in the business of their body and life, and that the most important relationship we will ever have is the one we have with our body. Our body is the most precious thing we own, and taking care of it is how we sustain ourselves.

I started taking care of my body when I stopped telling myself any kind of pain in my body and life were okay, and when I started to listen and communicate with my body, not bully it. I made the choice to be in a relationship with my body, and to use the sensation of pleasure to determine that the choices and decisions I was making were good for the whole me. I committed to a partnership with my body, until death do us part. This commitment has taken me closer to a healthy and happy, meaningful life, and a deeper connection to what is good and sustainable.

Along the way, I have discovered body and life essentials and non-essentials. At the top of my essentials list are good food, good people, good thoughts, good sleep, and dance. At the top of my non-essential list is worry, judgement, and overdoing and underdoing what needs to be done to keep me healthy and well.

Guided by the voice of the body, sensation, the choices and decisions I make are all intended to create pleasure; not the unhealthy, addictive kind of pleasure that leaves you feeling depleted, craving more, and needing more to feel good, but healthy pleasure. Healthy choices always make me feel good, better, and are accompanied by a deep sense that "this is right for me, this is good for me and my body." They leave me satisfied, and with a sense of calm and peace in my body, mind, emotional being and spirit.

Likewise, Michele is also in the business of body and life. She has developed a relationship with her body and in this book, rightfully takes her place among leaders dedicated to making us healthier and, yes, happier. Michele offers what I call simple ways to bestow "small acts of kindness" to your body and life. She shows us how to not only put good food and good nutrition inside our body, but to put good thoughts, good movement, good sleep, good feelings and a daily dose of dance in us to sustain our health and well-being. Michele encourages you to get out of your head, listen to your intuition and develop your awareness, as it relates to feeding your body, mind and soul.

As I read this book, I felt as if Michele was having a conversation with me, speaking authentically from her heart about her experience of living in a body, offering helpful tips, while simultaneously incorporating the science of nutrition and healthy movement. Michele does not lay out a strict regiment to follow, but instead encourages you to make choices to lead a balanced, joyful life. There's more than meets the eye with these simple, easy to follow suggestions. You don't need to know about nutrition or dance to reap the rewards from this book. All you need is the willingness to feel better. The rest is simple!

Introduction

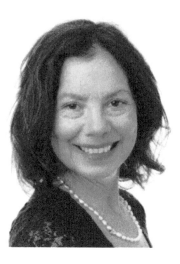

It's never too late to take charge of your health. I have noticed that even small changes can make a big difference. We all want to feel our best, especially as we age. And it's what you do every day that matters, not what you do from time to time. Day in, day out, consistent action to increase your vitality and boost your immune system means that the occasional 'less than optimum treat', such as a really late night, or a special cake with coffee, is fine, more than fine, if it feeds your soul. And you may notice that how you choose to feed your soul changes, the more healthy you become. ***More on 'feeding your soul' in Chapter 13, 'Chocolate Revealed!' and in the 'SHINE' section.***

I have always been interested in health. I remember wandering into an alternative hippy-type wholefood shop in the seventies as a teenager, and being impressed by the sacks of beans and rice, the large tins of olive oil, the glass jars packed with herbs and spices, that unique earthy smell, and the cat sleeping on the top of a box in the corner. I was awakening to another way. Yet my interest in well-being and the human body led me firstly along a more conventional route to a degree in physiology with biochemistry, and a Masters in nutrition with a short spell in medical research at Oxford University.

It was during my late twenties, while teaching biology, science and health education in London schools, that I began to realise I could actually improve how I felt by what I ate and drank. I remember trying out no dairy or wheat for three weeks, and feeling incredible.

I will be giving you some ideas of foods to avoid and foods to add so that you too can feel incredible.

Much later when I had my three children, and seriously needed more energy just to keep up with them, my interest expanded even further. Their health came into the equation as well as my desire for more energy. *In this book, you will find ways to increase your energy by removing certain foods that drain your battery, such as refined sugar. You will also learn about foods that support your immune system and how daily exercise and "happiness" practices will impact your 'joi de vivre'!*

I am a 'work in progress'. You know the saying 'you are what you eat'? I like this one even more: 'you are what you digest and absorb.' *If you suspect that your digestion and gut bacterial population (microbiome) is less than optimum, you'll be glad to know I will be expanding on this in Chapter 9, 'Fermented Foods and Probiotics'.* As a result of a few simple changes that I made and will share with you, my digestion and elimination has greatly improved; I feel better and look so much better too.

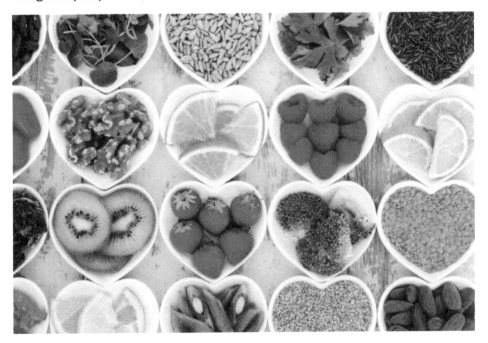

In the last 10 years, a combination of optimum nutrition and lots of exercise, particularly Nia, holistic fitness and also daily walks, I have been able to effortlessly and permanently drop two dress sizes. So again, I repeat, it is never too late!

People often say to me how well I look and also how 'good' I am at keeping to a healthy diet, as well as all the other things I do, to look after my well-being. Yes, I do a lot of great stuff (which I am excited to be sharing with you in this book), but quite frankly sometimes I think to myself, "How the heck do they know what I do!" and, "If only they knew about the chocolate and the coffee!" Naturally, people do make assumptions given that they see how passionate I am about a green and healthy lifestyle. But I am one of these people who needs to pay good attention to my well-being. If I don't, my body soon lets me know! I envy those who can eat and drink anything, go to bed at any hour, have tons of vitality, and still look great. Unfortunately, there are some people you and I know who have done this and it did not work out too well for them.

My focus is on **_prevention_** to avoid having to wade through a complicated and often frightening process of looking for a cure. I am constantly exploring, learning, researching and experimenting on myself, members of my family, friends, clients and Nia students who feel inclined to join me. What I recommend I have always tried out myself first. I am aware that we are all different, all unique, and it is important to discover what works for you. Become what Nia founder Debbie Rosas calls a 'Sensation Scientist'; sense what works for you, sense what makes you feel good, clear-headed, makes you feel better, what makes you come alive and feel happy – **_the Feel Better Factor._** If you would like to have a few quick tools at your fingertips to feel energised and happy, to set yourself up for the day with enthusiasm, if you would like to find peace and pleasure in food, I will offer some ways.

As you read *Eat Dance Shine*, imagine we are sitting across from each other at my kitchen table, chatting. Hopefully this will make it easier for you to absorb and then put some ideas into practice! At the end of the day, what you eat is a personal choice and it is important to find your own way, inform yourself, make your choices and then respect them. I am sharing with you my journey and I want to emphasise *I'm not saying you should do as I do*. Throughout this book, I hope you will take what appeals, what feels good in your body, your head, your heart, and make it your own. You are totally unique.

Writing this book has been amazing for my health; it has made me focus sharply on what I do, how I do it and why I do it. In fact, it's encouraged me 'to walk my talk'. And don't we all need reminding from time to time. So I want to thank you, the reader, for being here, ready to receive what I have to say. I hope this book will be interesting, entertaining, even inspiring, but more than anything, I hope that you will be motivated to take action today and start to develop new habits, make them your own, and experience the vibrant and abundant well-being you deserve.

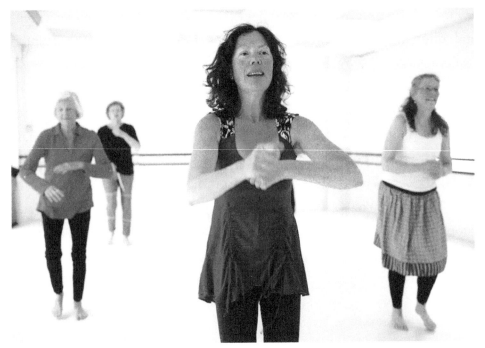

SECTION 1: EAT

Chapter 1
Dietary Dogma versus Freedom

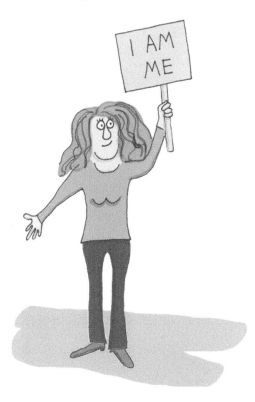

What we eat is a personal issue, whether we are talking about taste, health, emotions, religion, or ethical and environmental issues. The more you think about your health and the health of the planet, the more conscious you become, and the more choices you have to make.

Health is more important than any idealistic dietary dogma, be it Veganism, Raw Foodism, Paleo, Pegan (Paleo-Vegan), Low Fat, Mediterranean or Macrobiotic. At all times, the diet must serve you. I think it's best not to give yourself any labels; you eat food and what you eat varies over the course of your lifetime.

We are all different, and yet not so dramatically different; we are all human. Most experts agree that lots of vegetables are good for you; no one has ever said, "Just watch your vegetable intake!" Many natural health practitioners around the world recommend a plant-based diet i.e. 50-75% of your food coming from plants.

If you are reading this book, you are already likely to be pretty clear of the health problems associated with eating highly processed convenience foods, anything your great-great-grandmother would not have recognised as food. The question of eating meat is less clear and can be controversial. Not all meat is created equally. If you are eating meat too often and from unhappy, unhealthy animals, this can reduce your health, affecting you physically and, if you care to think about it, also on a psycho/socio/spiritual basis.

If eating meat feels good for your body and your general sense of well-being, then I believe that has to be respected. Keeping the level of meat consumption to an optimum level is an individual decision, but generally best in moderation i.e. not with every meal nor even every day; maybe three times a week.

How about making plants your main dish and animal products your side dish? I also recommend that the meat you choose is organic or wild as it will contain far fewer toxins from herbicides, pesticides and artificial fertilisers. From an ethical perspective, the animal will have had a more natural free-range existence.

An ideal way to improve digestion of animal products is to follow a simple and easy type of food combining:

- eat protein (meat/fish/eggs) with non-starchy vegetables (generally leafy and green, but also others such as onions, garlic, cauliflower and carrots)

- eat carbohydrates – grains and starchy vegetables (potatoes, beans, as well as grains such as rice, quinoa, buckwheat, millet, amaranth) with non-starchy vegetables.

BUT don't eat meat and carbohydrates in the same meal. Following this guideline, you are likely to notice an improvement in your digestion, reduced bloating and increased energy levels.

After many years of research and experimentation, I have developed a sense of what food is right for me, and what works. It has eventually become an intuitive process. I encourage you to do the same, to help you decide what is best for you. In other words, "awaken your inner guru".

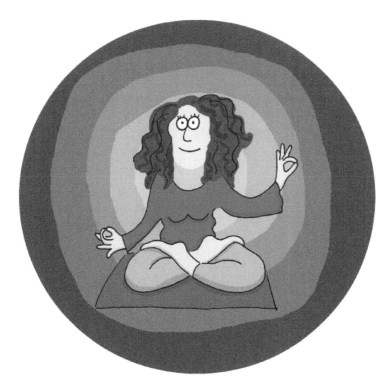

Exercise 1
To deepen your connection with your 'inner guru'

The 'Body Sway'

The Set-up:

Start by standing and holding a glass of water and silently ask your body, "Is this what I need right now?" Allow your body to sway very slightly forwards or backwards. Whichever way you sway while holding a glass of water means "Yes" (for most people, this is forwards).

The Test:

Now take any chosen piece of food or drink, and do the same process; you can even close your eyes to connect more deeply with your body's intuition. Now ask your body if it needs this food. Be spontaneous, without engaging the mind, and all you know about this food and your body. Notice the sway. Forwards is "Yes", meaning, right now, your body would benefit from eating the food you are holding. Backwards means "Not now".

Exercise 2
To develop awareness of what your body needs

You are asking your body's intuition, saying "Tell me what you need?" You may not get an answer to begin with, but that is fine. Remember that awareness is developed, without judgement. (Ref. 1)

Do this exercise in your kitchen, ideally, when no one else is around to disturb you.

It is best done when you are only mildly hungry. There are no right and wrong answers in this exercise. Just take the answers that come.

1. Choose any piece of food (e.g. a grape or a slice of cake)
2. Bring your awareness to the food in front of you
3. How hungry are you for it? On a scale of 0-10
4. Look at its shape, texture and colour
5. Smell the food
6. Now take a bite and slowly explore the sensations of the food in your mouth
7. Chew the food and notice how your mouth feels
8. Then swallow the food and notice how your mouth feels. Can you still taste the flavour?

9. How satisfied do you feel? On a scale of 0-10

10. How does your body feel? Notice any sensations

11. Do you want more of this food?

12. Is your body wanting more, or is your mind wanting more?

With practise, you will gradually be able to listen more easily to your body and what it needs. Try with many types of food and drink, and you will become more in tune.

Learn to listen to your body and sense how you feel. Being aware of how you feel after eating a meal is also useful. Notice if you feel:

- sleepy
- full of energy
- satiated, comfortable or bloated

Occasionally, I have started to cough or choke while eating something. I then stop and listen to my intuition, to see if that is a signal from my body to cease eating that food. I have even 'accidentally' knocked my hand and dropped the food before I could eat it. Is that a message? Listen to your wise body and your unconscious mind, and take note; make small changes, and your body will thank you. Learn from all your experiences.

My Story

Omnivore

I grew up as an omnivore, eating meat, dairy and way too much sugar while not giving it any thought at the time. A younger body is much more forgiving (except the teeth!) and able to process the good and the less than good diet, whereas later in life the body speaks more loudly about what it cannot tolerate. So like many young people, I did not give my diet much thought.

As a student, I went travelling during the summer with a close friend who was vegan. I watched how she ate and was fascinated, but not drawn to make, what seemed to me at the time, such radical changes. Later, I became interested in a more healthy wholesome organic diet, which still included meat and dairy. This evolved over the years, all the while adding more vegetables and fruit, and less processed food and less sugar.

Raw vegan

Fifteen years ago, I became very interested in a cleansing diet and the raw vegan food movement. I explored eating this way for several years, learning the value of green juices, carrot juice, wheatgrass juice, sprouts, nut milks, live fermented vegetables e.g. sauerkraut, as well as green smoothies, salads and delicious fruits. To this day, I make these foods and teach others how to make them and incorporate them into their diets. I believe an exclusively raw vegan diet is great for short periods of time to detoxify and support the body during healing (see Chapter 5 for more on juicing). These foods supply us with high nutrient levels and the smallest number of calories. But eating an exclusively raw food diet over a long period of time did not work for me. I found at times I was lacking in energy and continued to crave cooked dishes.

Nor has it worked for many others, causing some nutrient deficiencies and a lack of energy. It was an interesting episode and I learned many valuable techniques and recipes. I also learned a lot about myself and how much I love food, both raw and cooked.

I like to think of myself as open-minded, and as the economist John Maynard Keynes said "When the facts change, I change my mind. What do you do?" So I moved on.

Vegetarian

My journey then took me away from raw vegan to a vegetarian diet, including some carefully chosen animal products (ideally organic) such as:

- raw unpasteurised cow and goat's cheese
- free-range eggs
- live unsweetened yoghurt or homemade kefir

I was still not interested in returning to eating animals. Having read about the harrowing film *Earthlings*, which shows how animals are treated, reared and slaughtered, I decided that I could not eat farm-reared animals again. This is an individual and personal decision, made consciously. Unfortunately, in my opinion, too many people eat unconsciously, out of habit. It was once said:

> *"If abattoirs had glass walls, the eating habits of the human population would change to that of vegetarians overnight!"*

Nowadays, I love to eat a diet rich in raw vegetables, fruit, nuts and seeds, as well as wonderful freshly cooked vegetable dishes and occasionally dishes containing organic eggs or wild fish.

With an intention to reduce any perfectionist tendencies I may be brewing, from time to time I eat less than optimum food, such as a coffee and croissant. I love the following saying:

"The perfect is the enemy of the good."

It reminds me that trying to make something perfect can actually prevent me from making it just good.

Summary

- Avoid becoming attached to any one food ideology, and remain open-minded.
- If you eat meat and other animal food products, do so consciously. Make them organic and the side dish, rather than the main attraction.
- Adopt a simple food combining idea: meat (protein) plus vegetables or carbohydrate plus vegetables.
- Listen to your body's signals telling you:
    a. when you have eaten enough
    b. if you would benefit from avoiding a certain food.

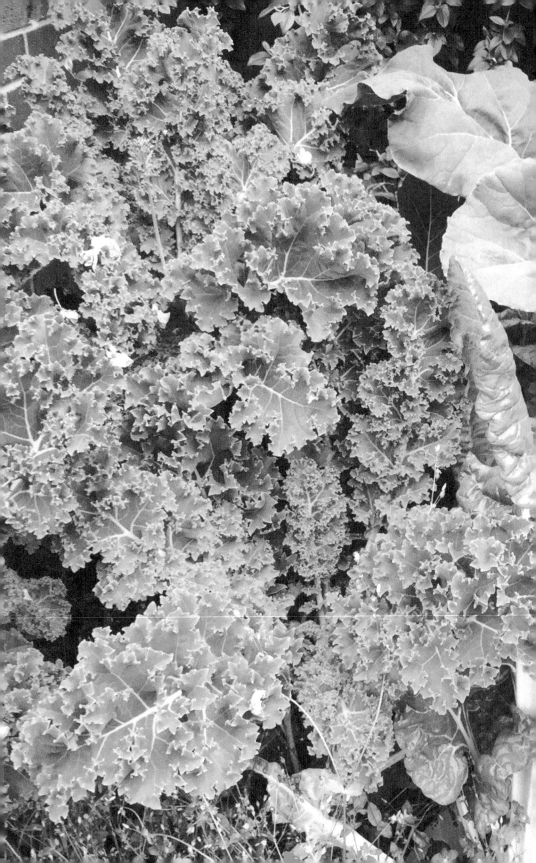

Chapter 2
Love Plants

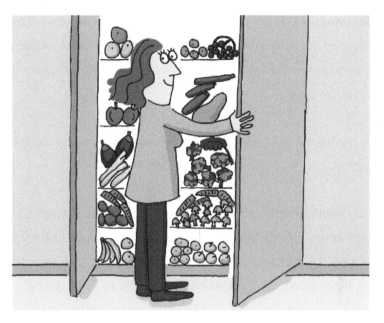

Every time you sit down to eat, you have a choice; to feed your immune system, or to feed a disease. Let's take a look at the benefits of eating more vegetables and fruits.

No one ever said to watch how many vegetables you eat. Yes, they said watch the fat, particularly fried foods, and to reduce sugar and salt, but never limit your vegetable intake. Why? Because by increasing the plant content of your diet, you are increasing the alkalinity of your body and this enables the body to carry out the remarkable processes that result in good health naturally – more energy, reduced stiffness and joint pain, improved digestion, better sleep, clearer thinking.

Michael Pollan, an American journalist, who describes himself as a "liberal foodie intellectual", puts it simply in his book *Food Rules: An Eater's Manual*: "Eat food. Not too much. Mostly plants."

An article (2013) in the *British Journal of Nutrition* describes a study using a fruit and vegetable puréed drink (FVPD) on 24 human subjects to test the protective antioxidant effects of a diet high in plants, especially in relation to heart disease. (Ref. 1) It's reassuring to know that they found an overall positive effect of drinking FVPD and affirms to me the value of home-made fresh juices and smoothies to increase absorption and bioavailability of the phytonutrients in plants.

As we age, we have a tendency to become more inflamed, hence the term 'inflammaging'.

Normally we think of inflammation as pain, redness and swelling such as, for example, when you sprain an ankle or cut your finger. Inflammation is the body's healing response, sending more blood to the area to initiate healing. It's how your immune system deals with an emergency.

But there is also a silent inflammation caused by a chronic overproduction of three hormones:

- Eicosanoids
- Insulin
- Cortisol

Need I say it, diet and stress are the main causes of this overproduction. You don't necessarily feel this silent inflammation, although it affects your heart, brain and immune system, and is linked to age-related chronic diseases such as arthritis, heart disease, colitis, even cancer. The good news is that with diet and lifestyle changes, inflammaging can be reduced, and it is possible to even reverse chronic diseases.

Also, as we age, we get less and less good at cellular housekeeping. We have 50 to 75 trillion cells to keep clean. When our body's ability to remove dysfunctional bits of protein in the cell (e.g. dead organelles and damaged proteins) reduces, then inflammation is stimulated. (Refs. 3 and 4)

Apparently we start aging as children! Quoting Christiane Northrup (who wrote *Women's Bodies, Women's Wisdom*) in a Hay House World Summit 2014 interview:

> *"Aging begins in childhood. In the Bogalusa Heart Study, they found the beginning of hardening of the arteries in six- and seven-year-olds ... well, we're aging, what, at fifty we start aging? At forty, we start aging? No. You start aging at eight!"*

A plant-based diet helps you to slow down 'inflammaging'. What I mean by a plant-based diet is when plants make up approximately 50-75% of your diet. If you choose to add animal products, this needs to be a much smaller percentage (20%), not necessarily daily, and of high quality i.e. organic, local and ethical.

An article called *Plant-Based Diets* in the journal *Nutritional Update for Physicians* in 2013 encourages physicians to recommend a plant-based diet to all their patients, especially those with diabetes, heart disease, high blood pressure and obesity, as a first-line treatment for chronic disease.

The plant-based diet maximises nutrient dense plant foods (lots of vegetables, cooked or raw, fruits, beans, seeds and nuts, in smaller amounts) while minimising processed foods, cooked oils and animal foods. (Ref. 2)

Like it or not, we cannot get away from inflammation as we age. But we can reduce it by including anti-inflammatory foods and superfoods. This is often referred to as an alkaline diet as it makes it easier for the body to maintain a slightly alkaline environment, with a blood pH of 7.35-7.45.

Plant foods contain phytonutrients, biologically active substances made by the plant which give them their colour, flavour and odour. Plants make them to protect themselves from pests, viruses, bacteria and excessive sunlight. Happily, they also happen to benefit humans when eaten.

Research shows that phytonutrients protect the human body from many ailments, including heart disease and certain cancers. There are hundreds, probably thousands, of phytonutrients in fruits, vegetables, grains and some herbs. These substances never exist in isolation in nature, e.g. vitamin C (ascorbic acid) occurs together with bioflavonoids, tyrosinase, and rutin, as well as other substances to form a complex group of synergistically interacting molecules. This explains why a whole food is generally better than an isolated supplement. See Chapter 10, 'Supplements'.

Fibre

Eating a plant-based diet will ensure that you are eating abundant amounts of fibre which helps to move food through your gut and keep your elimination process active.

Your body needs two different types of fibre:

- Soluble fibre from apples, blueberries, nuts and seeds.
- Insoluble fibre from dark green leafy vegetables, green beans, celery, carrots, and brown rice.

They help slow down your digestion and absorption, preventing a sharp rise in blood glucose. This means less sugar is stored at fat!

Soluble fibre also binds with cholesterol in the gut and prevents it being absorbed by the body, so helping to reduce cholesterol levels. Some foods, such as psyllium and flaxseeds, contain both soluble and insoluble fibre, and are especially valuable to take regularly.

A particular type of fibre called calcium glucarate found in both soluble and insoluble fibre (e.g. the skin of blueberries as well as cabbage and other brassicas) helps to keep oestrogen levels from rising too high. It binds to oestrogen molecules and then carries them out of the body via the colon.

The three top sources of fibre to add to your diet are:

- psyllium seeds
- linseeds (flaxseeds)
- brassica vegetables e.g. cabbage, broccoli, Brussel sprouts, kale, spring greens

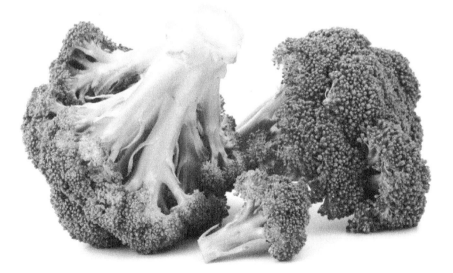

A word about fruit

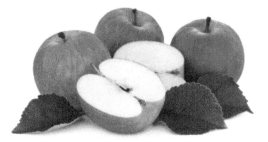

As you may be aware, the world of food and health is not without its contradictions, controversies and disagreements. Recently in certain circles, there has been a belief that fruit is not so healthy after all, due to its high sugar content. Along with this is the fashion for thinking that berries, grapefruit and lemons are fine, due to their low glycaemic index value.

Let's look at the sugar in fruit. Firstly, there is a huge difference between the naturally occurring fructose found in fruit (which is always present along with fibre, vitamins, minerals and antioxidants), and the purified isolated forms of sugar: sucrose (table sugar), corn syrup, glucose syrup, dextrose, maltose, glucose, fructose, high fructose corn syrup (HFCS) etc. that are added to cakes, biscuits, sweets, chocolates and sweetened drinks, not to mention most processed, packaged food.

Inspired by Professor J. Yudkin (in whose department I studied) who wrote *Pure, White And Deadly: How sugar is killing us and what we can do to stop it*, I am pondering how we got into this state of overkill with sugar. Looks to me like yet another direct consequence of the affluence, exploitation and greed of the major food multinationals over the last 100 years.

We know these purified, extracted sugars contribute hugely to the current epidemic of tooth decay, fatigue, diabetes, insulin resistance and obesity but less obvious in causing heart disease, cancer and/or even skin diseases such as seborrhoeic dermatitis. It is these sugar-laden beverages that enable people to consume huge excesses of calories. The normal satiety mechanisms of our bodies, that would regulate our intake, do not kick in, because of minimal fibre, but also possibly because refined sugar and HFCS are relatively novel foodstuffs, and so do not trigger this normal response, unlike when you consume fatty foods, proteins or even good old whole fresh fruit.

Many experts say that fruit in fact offers protection from these chronic diseases of affluence due to their high antioxidant and fibre content. Anthony William, author of *Medical Medium*, reminds us that the old saying was always, "An apple a day keeps the doctor away" not " An egg a day or a breast of chicken a day keeps the doctor away". He goes on to say "fruit has the power to heal disease, prevent it, sweeten our days, give us energy, and give us back our lives."

Only you will know which fruit feels good for you, how much, how often, and when. At the end of the day, I like to listen to my body rather than my head. I suggest you do the same.

Summary

Increase the plant content of your diet to 50-75%:

- reduce 'inflammaging'
- help maintain an alkaline environment
- ensure a rich supply of phytonutrients and fibre
- enjoy the fruit in a variety and quantity that suits your body best

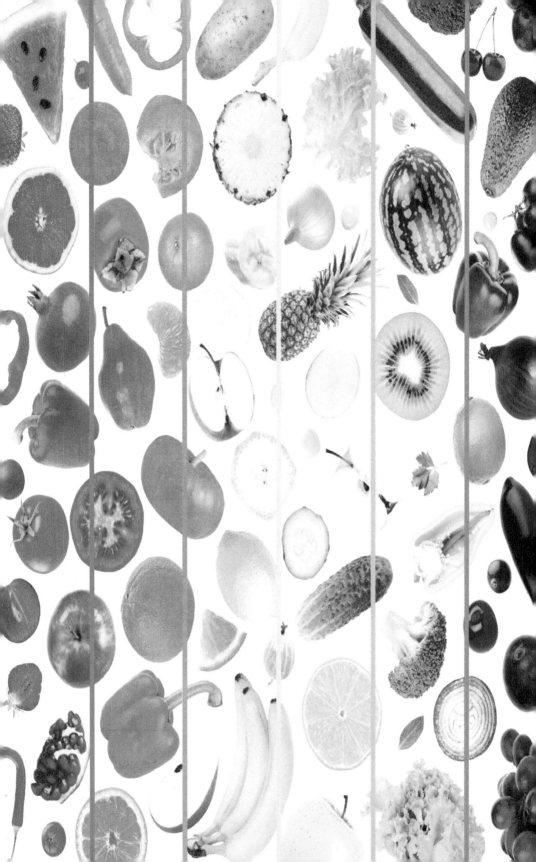

Chapter 3

Eat a Rainbow

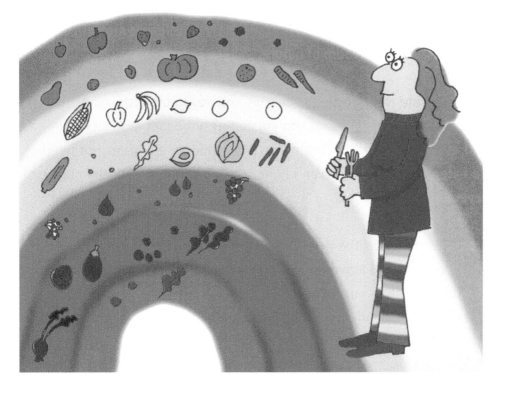

Imagine a gorgeous bowl of fruit and a basket of freshly picked vegetables, and notice the vibrant colours. This indicates an abundance of antioxidants.

An easy way to include more plant foods is to enjoy colour. I love to display all types of seasonal fruits and vegetables in bowls on my kitchen counter. They form an instant and wonderful decoration at the same time as reminding me and my family to eat plenty every day. Sometimes in the summer, I will leave a large plate of freshly washed, organic (even home-grown) strawberries in the middle of the table, instead of a vase of flowers, and the family can't keep their hands off them.

Berries provide red and blue phytonutrients, while green leaves provide chlorophyll rich in magnesium. Other vegetables and fruits provide yellow, orange and purple antioxidants. I like to remember that although we have identified and named these phytonutrients, there may well be hundreds, if not thousands, we have still yet to identify. This leaves me with a sense of wonder for the wisdom of nature.

Eating a wide range of different fruit and vegetable types and varieties increases the likelihood that you are getting abundant amounts of known and even unknown phytonutrients. This wide variety does not need to be eaten all in one day, even in one week, but rather over the course of several months or a year.

From ancient times, the days of the week have been linked to colours and the planets. Rudolf Steiner (mainly famous as a philosopher and creator of Waldorf Education and Biodynamic Farming) wrote about these colours, and their corresponding planets, organs of the body, days of the week, and how they impact us.

Exercise:

Colour guide

For a nourishing weekly rhythm, try using this table to identify the colour of the day and a reminder to eat plenty of that colour on the day. Even wearing that colour can be a fun reminder to yourself.

Monday	Tuesday	Wednesday	Thursday	Friday	Saturday	Sunday
Purple	Red	Yellow	Orange	Green	Blue	White
Moon	Mars	Mercury	Jupiter	Venus	Saturn	Sun
Brain/ reproductive organs	Gall bladder	Lungs	Liver	Kidneys	Spleen	Heart

So let colour be your inspiration and guide. Make colourful fruit and vegetable salads several times a week. It's also good to eat fruits grown locally and in season. However, I do love mangoes and bananas, and attempt to offset the environmental cost of their transport with other energy-saving measures in the house, rather than not eat them.

The Rainbow Diet by Chris Woollams is a valuable book for further inspiration and information on eating a rainbow of plant food.

Why berries?

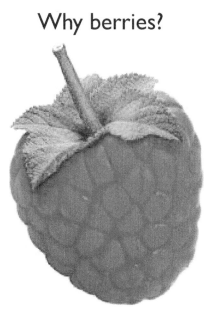

Berries may be considered a superfood as they are so rich in antioxidants, and are anti-inflammatory. Pink and red skins contain anthocyanins, which have been shown to be cancer fighting. (Ref. 5) A study in 1993 in Italy using bilberries showed an improvement in fibrocystic breast disease. (Ref. 6)

Blackberries are one of my favourites, packed full of nutrients, especially high in vitamin C, the mineral copper, fibre and the colourful, powerful antioxidant pigments lutein, zeaxanthin and beta-Carotene, which may play a role in slowing aging and age-related disease processes.

What's more, you can pick them yourself, wild and fresh. I love to eat them as I take a walk in nature.

Blueberries may reduce cortisol, the stress hormone, and are also very high in antioxidants. A recently published scientific paper said, "Daily blueberry consumption improves blood pressure and arterial stiffness in postmenopausal women with pre- and stage 1-hypertension." (Ref. 7)

Raspberries are full of antioxidants, especially organic raspberries, due to a greater level of anthocyanins. Unique to raspberries are the raspberry ketones, which may help with weight loss by increasing metabolism in fat cells. Studies are showing that raspberries also have anti-cancer benefits and help lower the risk of other diseases of chronic inflammation, such type 2 diabetes and atherosclerosis.

(See recipe Apple with Raspberry Super Sauce in Chapter 16)

Goji berries have been eaten in Tibet and other parts of Asia for thousands of years as a way of promoting longevity. In Tibet, they are called 'happy berries' as they help to deal with stress. They are particularly high in vitamin A and protein. See 'Resources' for where to buy them.

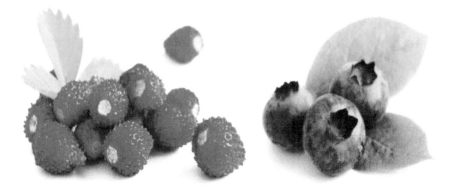

Recipe

'Berry tasty breakfast'

E at some berries today! And every day. Here's one of my favourites ways to eat berries.

Blend

- an apple or pear
- a banana
- 2 tbsp freshly ground linseeds
- a few tbsp water, if needed

(For a green option: add a large handful of baby spinach or ½ tsp spirulina powder)

Pour over a bowlful of berries (1-2 cups of berries – a mix of blackberry, raspberry, blueberry, strawberry)

Sprinkle with 1 tbsp soaked and rinsed seed mix (sunflower with pumpkin and sesame)

Dairy option:

Top with a few dollops of live (probiotic) unsweetened, natural yoghurt

Chocolate option:

Sprinkle with 1 tsp raw cocoa nibs

Pomegranates

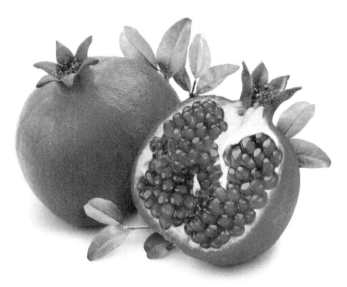

Vibrant red pomegranates may slow down the growth of breast cancer cells. (Ref. 9) Ellagitannins found in pomegranates inhibit the enzyme aromatase which normally converts androgen hormones to oestrogen, hence another way to reduce oestogens which can stimulate the growth of some types of breast cancer cells. Lowering oestrogen levels is usually desirable, as we tend to live in an oestrogen-polluted environment, meaning we are exposed to too much oestrogen.

How rainbow foods enhance eye health

Carotenoids are pigments and their colour ranges from pale yellow to bright orange through to deep red. Only two of the 600 carotenoid pigments in nature, namely lutein and zeaxanthin, are found in the retina (macula) of the eye. As the body cannot make these, we need to consume them daily for best eye health.

A study involving 4,000 people in 2013 (called *Age-Related Eye Disease Study AREDS2*) showed that if you already have macular degeneration (AMD), supplements containing lutein and zeaxanthin can slow the progression. They found that participants in the study whose diet was lowest in foods naturally containing lutein and zeaxanthin experienced the greatest benefit from taking daily supplements containing 10 mg/day of lutein and 2 mg/day for zeaxanthin. (Ref. 10)

Highest amounts of lutein and zeaxanthin are found in green leafy vegetables and to a lesser extent in other green or yellow vegetables, such as peppers. This confirms the benefit of eating plenty of greens, such as:

- raw and steamed spinach
- kale
- chard
- lettuces
- rocket
- watercress

For a wider variety of seasonal organic greens that the supermarkets don't stock, try Abel & Cole or Riverford.

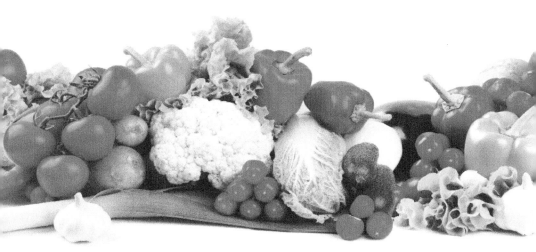

Colourful vegetables

Carrots and Carotenoids

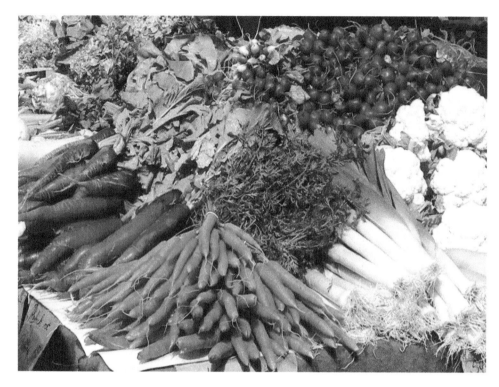

The most common carotenoid found in carrots that gives them their wonderful bright orange colour is beta-Carotene, a precursor to Vitamin A. This beta-Carotene, also in apricots, sweet potatoes, pumpkins, and other squashes, has been shown to reduce breast cancer risk when eaten regularly. (Ref. 10) Carotenoids are also present in green leaves such as kale and spinach, it's just that the green chlorophyll masks the yellow colour.

Interesting fact

Did you know that in autumn when leaves go yellowy-orange, it is due to the carotenoids that were present all along, becoming revealed as the green chlorophyll level in the leaf decreases?

Tomatoes and Lycopene

Another carotenoid, lycopene, is a powerful antioxidant abundant in tomatoes and goji berries. Interestingly, heat actually changes lypopene for the better, making it more easy for the body to absorb. Like other antioxidants, lycopene may play a role in preventing chronic diseases. (Ref. 11)

I personally won't be cooking all of my tomatoes, as there's nothing like my mother's simple raw tomato and red onion salad.

Recipe

Tomato and red onion salad

Mix

- 4 tomatoes, thinly sliced
- red onion, thinly sliced

Dress with olive oil, cider vinegar and sea salt to taste!

Onions and Quercetin

Quercetin occurs in a variety of brightly coloured foods and guess what? It has antioxidants and anti-inflammatory properties. Quercetin was shown to inhibit breast cancer growth in a Petri dish study in 2012 (Ref. 12).

The highest amount of quercetin is found in capers, which are the buds of the Capparis spinosa plant. Capers in olive oil can be bought in jars (Biona) and are delicious sprinkled onto a green leafy salad.

Other foods rich in quercetin are onions, red onions in particular and the fresher the better, but also in dark red and blue fruit.

Unlike lycopene, cooking significantly reduces the content of quercetin, another reason to use raw or only lightly cooked quercetin-rich fruits and veg. (Ref. 13)

Broccoli

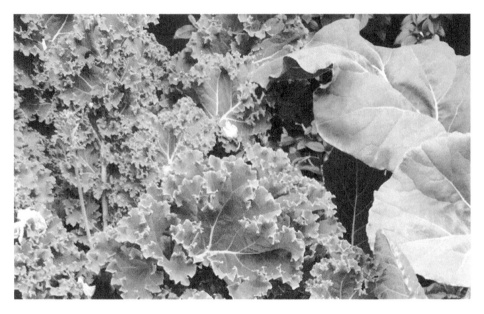

The wonderfully green broccoli and other brassicas (also called cruciferous vegetables), such as cabbage and Brussel sprouts, contain sulforaphane, a chemical that stimulates the body's natural ability to fight cancer, by preventing cancer cell growth and increasing the rate at which cancer cells commit suicide (apoptosis). It has been found that three-day-old broccoli sprouts contain up to 100 times more sulforaphane than that found in mature broccoli. You can easily grow your own broccoli sprouts in your kitchen.

It is also possible to now buy powdered and dried broccoli sprouts, which can be mixed into juices or smoothies (available from many sites online).

46

Some experts consider brocolli sprouts to be a top anticancer superfood! So all in all make broccoli and its relatives one of your best friends.

Geeky science alert

As if you need another reason to eat and juice your brassicas, they are rich in diindolylmethane (DIM). This plant chemical guides oestrogen breakdown in the liver, diverting it to the healthy pathway (2-hydroxy). This results in 'good' oestrogen metabolites that, when released into the bloodstream, help with the prevention of heart disease, the building of strong, healthy bones, and soft, supple skin.

Conversely the 'bad' oestrogen pathway (16-hydroxy) results in metabolites responsible for many of oestrogen's undesirable actions, including weight gain and an increased risk of breast and other gynecological cancers.

Oestrogen dominance is a consequence of living with oestrogenic pollution (see Chapter 14, 'Clean Living'), a weak liver, a stressful lifestyle, or as a result of normal aging. So it's really important to look after your liver. Liver-friendly foods to include are carrots, rocket, watercress and garlic.

Summary

- Become more aware of colour in fruits and vegetables, and eat a variety of colour each day to consume a wide range of phytonutrients.

- Use the table to follow the colours of the days of the week, if you want a reminder to eat different colours.

- Consider berries as a superfood, packed with anti- inflammatory nutrients. Eat locally grown berries when in season.

- Carotenoids found in yellow, orange and red foods, as well as green leaves, increase eye health.

- Eating tomatoes and onions provide more antioxidants (lycopene and quercetin, respectively) that may play a role in reducing and preventing chronic diseases.

- Brassicas, such as broccoli, provide sulforaphane that may stimulate the body to fight cancer, as well as containing DIM which may support the liver in reducing the level of circulating oestrogens.

- Pomegranates containing ellagitannins may be an aromatase inhibitor which slows down the production of oestrogens.

Chapter 4
Grapes and Wine

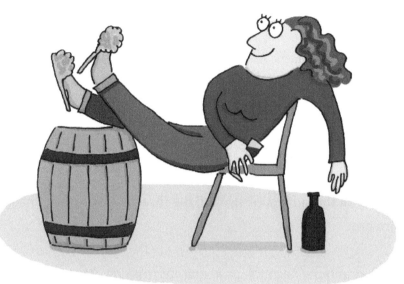

All grapes contain a mix of antioxidants, which are beneficial for a healthy heart as well as having anticancer properties. The most well-known one, resveratrol, is produced in the skin of red, purple and white grapes, to protect the grapes from fungal infection as they ripen in the sun.

Loaded with resveratrol, grapes are recommended for their demonstrated positive impact on cell health and longevity. There are many other phytonutrients (including beta-Carotene and fibre), not only in the skin but also in the pulp and seeds. So eat whole grapes, rather than grape juice!

As for wine and how much is okay, veer on the conservative side. After all, alcohol is a neurotoxin. Although for women past the menopause, it is thought that drinking a small amount of wine helps to protect against heart disease and stroke, the exact amount is not clear. So it's best not to kid yourself, and to keep a check on healthy limits.

I think it's wise to drink a maximum of four glasses of wine per week. The good news is that resveratrol is found in grapes and chocolate too!

Dr Mercola (Mercola.com and *New York Times* bestselling author) says:
"Although resveratrol is found in red wine, I can't recommend drinking wine regularly, in the hope of extending your life because alcohol is a neurotoxin that can poison your brain and harm your body's delicate hormonal balance. Instead, get your resveratrol from natural sources, such as whole grape skins and seeds, raspberries, and mulberries."

While we are on the subject of alcohol, the three main causes of hangover symptoms are:

- dehydration – alcohol is a diuretic making you pee more, taking water from the organs, including the brain which slightly contracts, resulting in a headache.

- alcohol metabolism bi-products (e.g. acetaldehyde).

- impurities (e.g. zinc and other metals) that have been added during fermentation; there's more in red wine and champagne, less in white wine, while vodka has the least.

One of the best hangover cure tricks is to drink a large glass of water, with a pinch of sea salt added, before going to bed. A fruit juice can also help as it provides the brain with nutrients. A few drops of milk thistle tincture in water may help in protecting the liver.

Then 'the morning after', a detoxifying and rehydrating juice is very effective.

A citrus juice will replace some of the lost vitamin C – 1 grapefruit, 2 oranges and 1/2 lemon.

Or try one of these juice combinations:

- 2 carrots, 1 apple, 2 sticks celery and a large handful of spinach
- 1 beetroot, 3 carrots and 2 oranges

Also see Chapter 5, 'The ultimate fast food - Juices'.

Summary

Grapes contain resveratrol, which may support the health of the heart and have anticancer properties. As alcohol is a neurotoxin, the consumption of wine to obtain resveratrol ideally needs to be kept to four glasses a week. Whole grapes and raspberries contain resveratrol too.

Hangover cures include drinking a large glass of water before sleep, and a large fresh vegetable and fruit juice on waking.

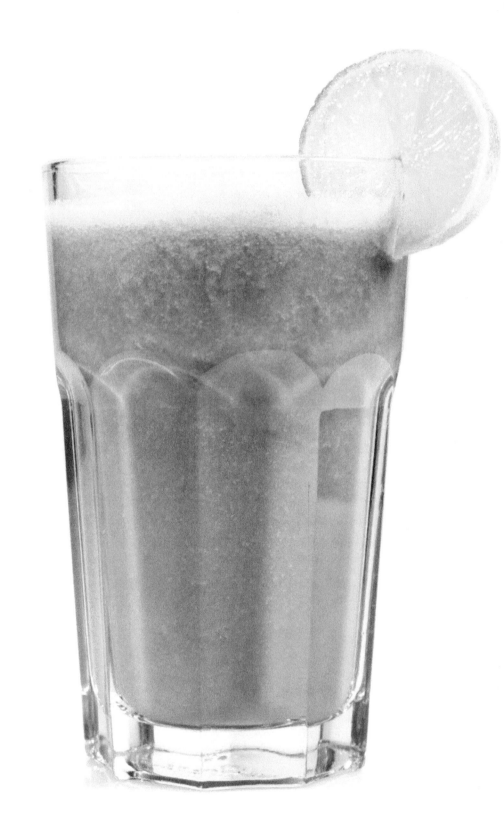

Chapter 5
The ultimate fast food - Juices

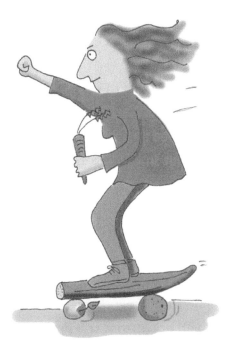

Why is juice a fast food?

Freshly made vegetable juice is a soothing and efficient way to get lots of nutrients into your body in a short time; and the absorption of nutrients is tremendous. Great to start the day right, with the balancing effect of a freshly made juice packed with bioavailable nutrients. It can help to reduce cravings, avoid the sinking feeling mid-morning, and generally start to improve your whole digestive system. It requires no or very little energy to digest, conserving energy for other activities.

Vegetable juicing is the single most effective holistic technique I practice daily, in the kitchen. I notice how vibrant I feel, the increase in my energy levels, and clear-headedness.

In *Vegetable Juicing for Everyone*, Dr Andrew Saul says:

> *"In the 39 years that I've been working with folks and teaching in the natural health arena, the one thing that's helped more people more consistently is vegetable juicing."*

Dr Saul was originally inspired by Max Gerson, who is famous for using juices to rid himself of migraines. Gerson later went on to develop the Gerson Therapy, which has helped thousands of people heal from advanced cancer and can be read about in *Healing the Gerson Way – Defeating Cancer and other Chronic Diseases* by Charlotte Gerson with Beata Bishop.

Thousands of cancer patients have visited the Gerson Institute in Mexico and Hungary, and similarly the Hippocrates Health Institute in Florida, benefiting hugely from the education and healing of the programmes they offer. Although not the same, both programmes emphasise the importance of learning how to make and drink large amounts of vegetable juice and live entirely on plant-based foods to cleanse and heal.

Why not just eat the vegetables?

Well it's not possible to consume that volume of vegetables, whether it's carrots, celery or kale, in one go. By removing the fibre, you can consume a large volume of vegetables. And as long as the whole food you eat on a daily basis gives you plenty of fibre, then there is no problem removing it when making vegetable juices.

Dr Saul says:

"The advantage of the juicer is, first of all, it reduces large amounts of vegetables into a few manageable glasses. That means you get a nice, easy-to-take, and quick food concentrate."

Needless to say, use organic produce wherever possible and peel the skin off, if using non-organic produce. To balance the bitter taste of some leafy vegetables, I like to use half a lemon or lime, with peel, or half to one apple. It's good to explore and experiment until you find what works for you. The main thing is to juice every day!

When it comes to fruit, it is best eaten, chewed and savoured whole rather than juiced. Use fruit juices as an occasional treat. When juiced, all the fibre is removed and the release of fruit sugars is accelerated, causing too large a sugar spike, with an increased insulin surge.

The time it takes to make the juice is short. However, the time it takes to clean the juicer, to be honest, can be tedious. I think of it as a worthwhile investment in my health, and often make use of the time to listen to something inspiring and informational.

Juicing really is for everyone. Even people with irritable bowel syndrome, Crohn's disease, and other kinds of gastrointestinal problems can usually handle vegetable juice, whereas they may not be able to easily eat a lot of raw vegetables. Cabbage juice is particularly good for the gut.

In his film *Super Juice Me!*, Jason Vale gave large amounts of cabbage juice to one of the participants who had colitis, with great results.

Here's the recipe:

Jason Vale's Cabbage Juice

- 1/2 head of red cabbage
- 2 apples
- 3 inches of cucumber
- big lump of ginger (optional)

Jay Kordich, with Dr Garnet Cheney, healed stomach and duodenal ulcers (Ref. 1) in patients, who were prisoners on Alcatraz Island, within 14 days, but more often in just two to three days. They drank four cups a day (approximately 1 litre) of this juice:

The 3 C Juice
(freshly made, as it does not store well)

Juice:
- Cabbage – preferably green (as it contains glutamic acid)
- Carrot and celery – small amounts of both to make it palatable

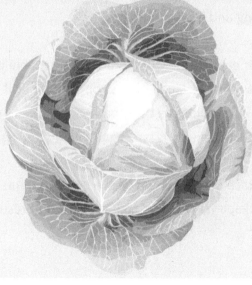

Mega Green Vegetable Juice

This is a serious drink, with an interesting lemon and ginger twist. To make your juice more appealing as a vegetable juice beginner, you can start with more apple and less leaves, until your taste adjusts. I sometimes say to folks, "Don't worry about liking it; that will come later. Just regard it as your medicine and knock it back!"

Juice:
- ½ cucumber, chopped
- 2 sticks celery, chopped
- a large handful of greens e.g. kale, chard, dandelion, nettle, spinach, wheatgrass, rocket, lettuce, parsley
- ½ -1 inch ginger
- ½ lemon, with peel
- ½ inch fresh turmeric root (optional)
- ½ apple (optional)

Boost - to increase the absorption of fat-soluble nutrients like beta-Carotene and turmeric, before drinking add and stir in one of the following:
- ¼ cup of almond milk, or
- 1 tbsp olive oil/coconut oil, or
- blend with half an avocado – this wonderful fruit is high in monounsaturated fats.

Interesting fact

In case you dislike ginger, it's worth cultivating a liking for this ancient spice! A research study in 2012 showed that a crude extract of ginger (Zingiber officinale) inhibited the proliferation of breast cancer cells, without significantly affecting the viability of non-tumour breast cells. (Ref. 2) See Chapter 12, 'Superfoods'.

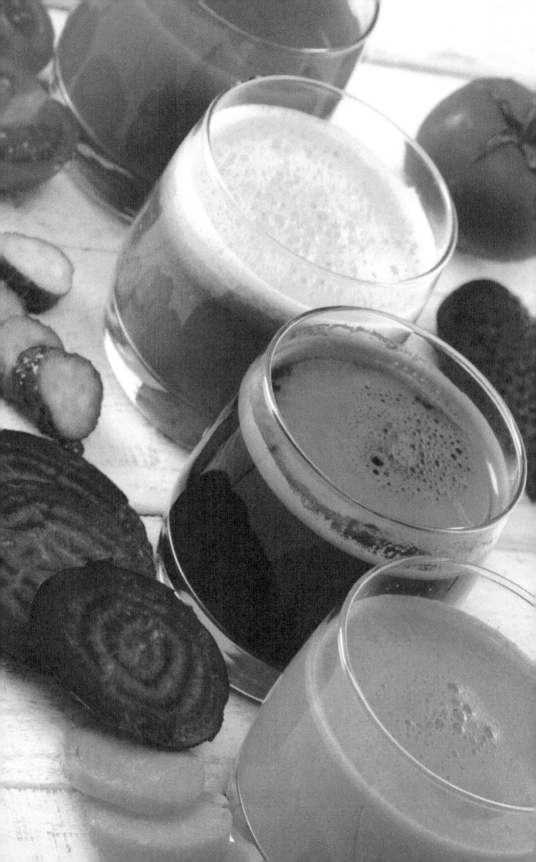

Meal in a glass

This recipe adds hemp milk to the juice, making it more of a meal.

Juice:
- 500g carrots
- 2 apples
- ½ cucumber
- ½ lemon
- large handful of curly kale or chard
- 1 inch piece of ginger

Pour the juice into a blender jug and add:
- a large handful of spinach
- ½ -1 glass freshly made hemp milk. (See Chapter 6, 'Nuts and Seeds' for recipe 'Hemp milk')

Blend and enjoy!

Gerson's carrot juice

Eight glasses of this juice are drunk each day on the Gerson Therapy!
Another favourite of mine for its simplicity:

Juice:
- 4-5 carrots
- 1 green apple (optional)

The Gerson Institute says that if you are healthy, it is fine to mix this juice with other vegetables, green and red. However, if working with the full Gerson Therapy for aiding in healing a chronic disease, it is important to keep the carrot and apple juice as described previously.

Interesting facts

- Did you know that vegetable juice qualifies as part of your water intake for the day?

- The water in vegetables is 'structured' or 'energised' by being in the living plant, and may have more health promoting qualities than other water.

How long does juice keep?

The best practice is to make the juice and drink it immediately. If this is not possible, firstly keep it cool. Then to minimise nutrient loss by oxidation, it's important to store the juice in a lidded jar (ideally glass), filling it right to the top, to reduce air contact, and pop it in the fridge. Always drink the same day! And if for any reason you don't, throw it on the compost heap. Why? Well Dr Mercola explains that methanol (methyl alcohol), which is normally bound to pectin in vegetables and fruit, and leaves the body along with the fibre, actually dissociates in the juice.

The longer juice is stored, the more free methanol it contains. On drinking the old juice, methanol enters the blood stream. Unlike other mammals, our human body cannot deal with methanol and break it down to harmless formic acid. Studies are starting to reveal that methanol (often released from aspartame) is linked to the development of Alzheimer's. (Ref. 3)

What is the best way to juice?

Firstly, whatever juicer you have is 'best'; the main thing is to just start using it! Later on when you have developed a new habit or are back in the habit, you can decide whether to upgrade and invest in another juicer. If you are new to juicing, then it does depend on your budget. Here are two of the most common types of juicers, plus a third method that does not require a juicer:

1. The cheapest is the centrifugal juicer that uses a spinning process with tiny blades to shred and separate the fibre. These juicers are quick and easy to use and clean. However, the pulp is quite damp, so less efficient at extracting the juice. Dr Saul estimates you could be getting 20-25% less juice from the centrifugal juicer. Another disadvantage is that it does not juice green leaves very well, nor wheatgrass.

2. The single gear or twin gear (masticating juicers) chew up the vegetables and pushes them through a strainer. This method is much more efficient, resulting in a drier pulp. They can cost up to four times more than the centrifugal juicer. However, over time, it saves money as you get more juice for less vegetables. I use a single gear also known as a 'slow juicer', as the low-speed rotation greatly reduces oxidation and therefore preserving the enzymes. This results in the juice staying fresher for longer.

No juicer? Another way!

There is a third method that I also like to use, involving a blender and a nut milk bag (or a fine sieve). A Vitamix blender, with its large two-litre jug, works a treat, but any high-powered blender will be great. I fill the jug with chopped vegetables, making sure the high water content vegetables are at the bottom near the blades, green leaves on top.

Blend until all the vegetables are liquidised, and strain into a glass bowl or jug using the nylon nut milk bag or fine seive. Squeezing the bag with your hands makes sure that the pulp is dry, even drier than pulp produced with a centrifugal juicer. There are serious 'juice feasters' who exclusively use this method every day for their entire juice 'feast', which can be up to 92 days! The juice feasting concept, created by David Rainoshek, is a diet consisting exclusively of juices, mainly green vegetable).

Summary

- Juice is a super 'fast food' as it's easy to consume, digest and absorb, providing concentrated nutrients to the body.

- Vegetable juice consumption is possibly the most effective daily kitchen and health habit to practice.

- Use organic vegetables and fruit wherever possible.

- Cabbage juice is particularly beneficial for the gut.

- Lemon and ginger, as well as a small amount of apple, juiced with green vegetables, make it more palatable.

- Adding a small amount of fat e.g. 1 tbsp olive oil or coconut oil, increases the absorption of fat soluble nutrients.

- Drink the juices as soon as possible and on the same day to minimise nutrient loss and prevent consumption of methanol.

- Use whatever juicer you have; the main thing is to get started and keep juicing. Once you are in the habit of juicing, decide what type of juicer suits you best.

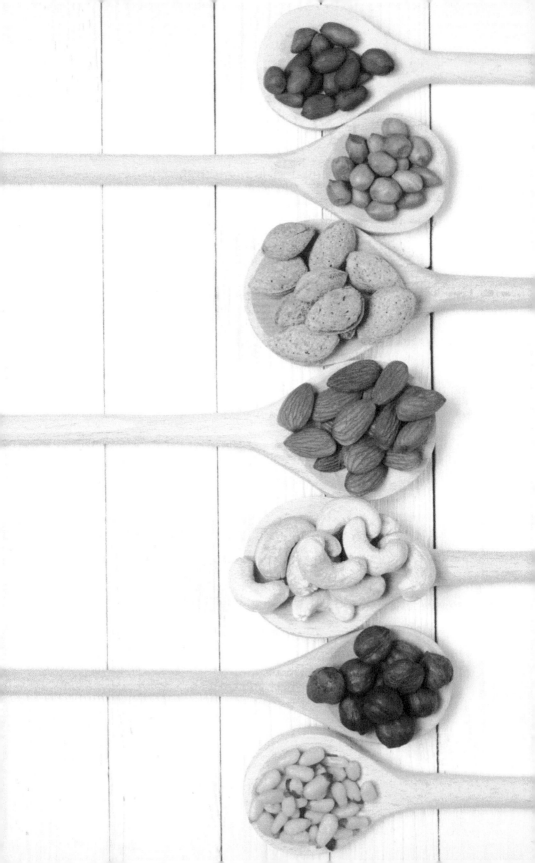

Chapter 6
Nuts and Seeds

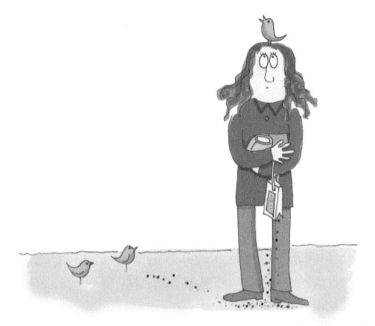

I heard this joke donkey's years ago, and for some reason it has stuck with me. "Why did the squirrel float downriver on his back? To keep his nuts dry!" Unlike the squirrel, who was probably carrying fresh nuts straight off a tree, the nuts most available to us are dried nuts. I recommend you avoid eating dry nuts (and that includes roasted and salted, apart from as a rare treat). When in this dormant dry condition, the water content is so low that not much can live off them, even moulds and bacteria. Dry nuts and seeds are also hard to digest, as they contain an enzyme inhibitor, which, in nature, stops the nut from germinating, until conditions are right for successful growth. This enzyme inhibitor also blocks our digestive enzymes, hence making the nuts hard to digest. Humans, unlike sheep and cows, cannot digest phytic acid, and as it binds to minerals (especially iron and zinc) in our food, it prevents their absorption. The tannins present in the nut/seed coat are antimicrobial. However, views about whether tannins are harmful vary.

Soak your dry nuts and seeds

The benefits of soaking nuts and seeds:

- removes the enzyme inhibitor.
- the nut (in most cases) will begin its process of germination (as long as it has not been previously killed by roasting and salting), and this activating process may make the nutrients more bioavailable, i.e. easier to digest and absorb.
- removes phytic acid and tannins (hence the brownish colour in the soak water) .

Soak your nuts and seeds overnight, in some filtered water, enough to cover them well. Drain and rinse the next day and store these activated nuts for up to four days in the fridge. They may well not last that long due to being so popular; they will get eaten! My favourites are almonds, hazelnuts and sunflower seeds.

So what's great about nuts and seeds?

Nuts are a dense food: high in fat, hence the calories, as well as containing protein, fibre (highest in almonds), vitamin E and B1, magnesium, copper and manganese. They also contain resveratrol, that wonderful phytonutrient present in red grape juice, red wine and also chocolate. Nuts and seeds are packed with healthy fats; walnuts contain more omega 3 fatty acids than any other nut.

The fat content can make you feel quite full and satiated after eating a handful. Overeating on nuts can be tough on the digestion and cause more calories to be consumed than you may need or like. Most days, it is sufficient to limit your intake to one handful. If you are concerned that you love nuts too much and you will overeat on them, a little tip: just make sure you have a small amount every day and that binge mentality, with respect to nuts, will soon fade, knowing that it is not your last chance to ever again eat nuts.

Recipe

Easy-going Nut Roast

A chapter on nuts would not be complete without a Nut Roast recipe. Here's one I created from about six other recipes, taking bits I like from each. Feel free to be creative and flexible with different nuts and amounts.

Note that the onion is not fried in oil but simmer-fried in ½cm water. See Chapter 8 – 'To cook or not to cook?' for more details.

Simmer-fry the first four ingredients in ½cm water for three minutes.

- 1 stick celery
- 1 red pepper
- 1 red onion
- 2 cloves garlic

Add, and heat for a minute, the following:
- 1 tbs olive oil
- 1 tsp oregano
- 1 tbs tomato puree

Mix and heat for one further minute:
- 6 brazil nuts, chopped
- handful almonds and handful cashews, grinded

Add all the nuts to the pan with:

- 1 tbsp sunflower seeds
- 1 tbsp sesame seeds
- 2 tbsp of chia seeds
- ½ vegetable stock cube and enough water to make a thick dough

Add 1 tbsp olive oil and mix well. Simmer on low heat for 5 mins.

Season to taste and press down in an oiled baking loaf tin.

Heat in medium oven (approx 180C) for 20-30 mins until a brown crust forms on top. Remove and cool before slicing. Goes well with onion gravy and a green salad.

Linseeds

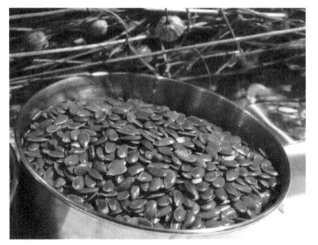

Linseeds (also called flaxseed) contain a high amount of both soluble and insoluble fibre, great for bowel health. They are also a good source of healthy fats – omega-3 fatty acids (1.8 grams of plant omega-3s per tablespoon of ground linseed). Finally, they are by far the richest source of lignans, a plant oestrogen, also found in smaller amounts in many vegetables, fruits, wholegrains, nuts and other seeds.

What are lignans and why are they important?

Lignans are a form of plant oestrogen (phytoestrogen) which, once eaten, are converted to an active form by gut bacteria (another reason to protect these bacteria by avoiding unnecessary use of antibiotics). As many breast cancers (and some forms of prostate cancer) are stimulated by oestrogen i.e. oestrogen-positive, you can benefit from consuming these plant oestrogens as they block or reduce the action of human oestrogen. In this way, lignans from linseed can protect against hormone-associated breast cancer.

The best way to take organic linseeds and get the most out this tiny golden-brown seed is to grind them yourself. If you purchase pre-ground linseeds, the fats are more likely to be oxidised (rancid), doing more damage than good. Likewise to prevent oxidation, grind your linseeds just before you eat them; it's no good doing a large batch for the week.

Grind two to four tablespoons of linseeds (flaxseeds) daily and mix into your cereal, porridge, smoothie, juice, or sprinkle on your vegetable dish or soup. I use a small coffee bean grinder that I keep especially for this purpose, but a Nutribullet works well too.

Linseed oil can also be used, though it must be kept in the fridge, and never used in cooking, as the omega-3s are vulnerable to temperature and light.

Psyllium seed husks are also a great source of soluble dietary fibre. One teaspoon can be stirred into a juice, once a day, to prevent constipation and keep a healthy colon.

Nut butters are a nutritious and useful spread for those moments between meals, or for picnics.

Some say peanut butter is best avoided, as peanuts (which are not actually nuts but belong to the legume family) are prone to a fungal infestation producing a lethal aflotoxin. However, in the decades that I have been buying peanut butter for my family, this has never been a problem. Almond and hazelnut butter, as well as pumpkin butter, are tasty and nutritious alternatives.

Here's some afternoon snack ideas that are so much better than reaching for the packet of crisps or slice of cake:

- Apple slices dipped in nut butter
- An apple with a handful of soaked and rinsed nuts
- Nut butter spread on rice cakes, or bread topped with thin slices of cucumber or tomato

Nut and seed milks

Nut and seed milks are a wonderful alternative to dairy milk. Many people are intolerant to dairy milk (and cheeses) without even knowing it, and feel much better when leaving them out of their diets. There are many nut milks now commercially available in cartons in the supermarkets, but a word of caution: they will be pasteurised so contain less available nutrients, and can contain added sugar and artificial flavourings. Making your own nut and seed milks will provide you with a far more nutritionally superior drink, and you can choose how to flavour it. Making your own can seem daunting at first, but I cannot emphasis enough how simple and quick they are to make. They store well in the fridge for up to three days.

My favourites are almond and hemp milk.

Recipe

Almond milk

(or substitute the almonds for hazelnuts, brazil or cashew nuts)

* Soak 1 cup of nuts overnight in 2 cups of water.

* Drain and rinse thoroughly the following morning.

* Blend in a high-speed blender/liquidiser 1 cup of nuts with 1 cup of water.

Options:

* For a thicker, creamier milk, use ½ cup of water.

* For a sweeter milk, add 1 de-stoned, chopped medjool date to the blender.

* Finally, pour into a nut milk bag (these nylon bags can be bought online) and squeeze out the milk into a bowl or jug. You can also pour the liquid through a fine mesh sieve and allow the milk to drip through.

What to do with the almond pulp?

If you are short of time, it can be added to your compost heap.

Otherwise, try one of these almond pulp recipes.

Gluten-free Banana and Almond Muffins
– with vegan options

Ingredients

2 ripe bananas

2 eggs, or vegan egg replacement powder (Orgran – no egg)

3 tbsp sweetner e.g. coconut palm sugar, agave nectar, maple syrup, barley malt syrup, date syrup or honey

3 tbsp unsweetened almond milk

1 tsp pure vanilla extract

1 tsp baking powder

1 cup almond pulp

½ cup oat flour (ground oats) or buckwheat flour

Optional toppings: chopped nuts, rolled oats

Instructions

- Preheat oven to 180°C and lightly oil a muffin tray.
- In a large bowl, beat the eggs or prepare the egg replacement powder following instructions.
- Next, add the bananas and mash. Add agave, baking powder, vanilla, almond milk and stir.
- Add the almond pulp and oat flour, and stir once more. Taste to see if it needs more sweetener.
- Bake for 25-34 minutes, or until a toothpick inserted into the centre comes out clean and they become firm to the touch.
- Remove from oven and cool for 5 minutes. Then place on cooling rack, until they become more firm.
- Enjoy!

There are many other online recipes for baking with almond pulp.

For ideas that do not involve baking:

Almond Hummus

Mix:

- 1 cup dry almond pulp
- ¼ cup tahini
- 1 clove of garlic, crushed
- 1 tsp lemon juice or apple cider vinegar
- 4 tsp olive oil
- ¼- ½ cup water
- ½ tsp salt
- ground coriander and cumin (optional)

Top with diced olives, tomatoes, onions and drizzle with olive oil. Finally, sprinkle with sumac.

Almond balls

Mix well by hand or food processor:
- 1 cup shredded coconut
- 6-12 dates, not soaked, chopped finely
- 1 banana, mashed
- ¼ cup coconut oil
- 1 cup almond pulp

By hand, form into balls and roll in raw cocoa powder or sesame seeds.

Recipe: Hemp milk

Soak 1 cup hemp seeds overnight, rinse and drain as with the nuts. Add 1 de-stoned, chopped medjool date and a small piece of vanilla bean. Blend and strain. Almond milk and hemp milk can be used as a drink, added to recipes, poured over cereals, and makes a wonderful latte.

Energy Boosting Tip
from Pauline Mostyn
Matcha Green Tea Almond Latte

Make a green tea using this delicious recipe for a morning lift!

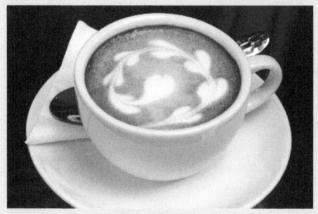

- ¼-½ teaspoon Matcha green tea powder
- ¼ cup freshly made almond milk
- ¾ cup hot water
- Add ¼-½ teaspoon Matcha green tea powder to your blender.
- Add freshly boiled water (remember when blending hot water it's important to leave a good amount of room at the top of the jug).
- Add approx. 20 ml almond milk and blend. Pour into a mug, adding the froth on top! Enjoy!

Summary

- Avoid eating nuts and most seeds in their dry form. Instead, pre-soak overnight and rinse them.

- Removing the enzyme inhibitor and phytic acid in nuts and seeds and activating the nut/seed makes the nutrients more bioavailable.

- Nutrient dense, nuts and seeds contain fat, protein, fibre, some vitamins and many minerals.

- Linseeds are a valuable source of fibre for bowel health, omega-3 fatty acids and phyto-oestrogens.

- Grind linseeds daily (2-4 tbsp) and consume as soon as you have ground them.

- Use nuts and nut butters as a snack.

- Nut and seed milks are a great alternative to dairy milk. Making your own is simple.

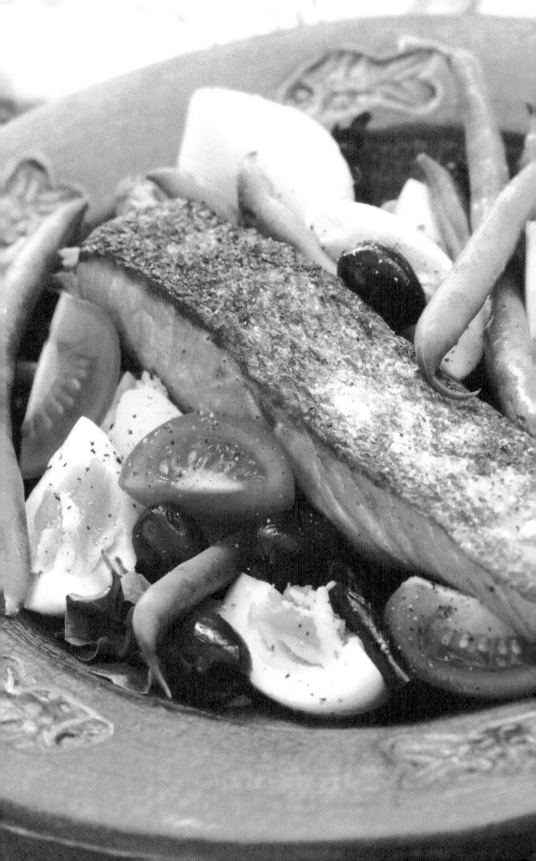

Chapter 7
Fatty Fishy Facts

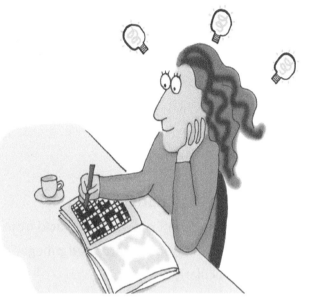

The subject of healthy fats can be confusing, and there's much talk about the importance of omega-3 fatty acids, essential fatty acids and fish oils. I will attempt to lay this out clearly so that you can then make some informed choices.

What are essential fatty acids?

There are only two that are 'essential', meaning they must be provided by your diet as your body cannot make them itself:

1. Linoleic acid (LA, omega-6, 18:2w6) – found in leafy vegetables, seeds, nuts, grains and vegetable oils, such as sunflower, safflower and evening primrose.
2. Alpha-linolenic acid (ALA, omega-3, 18:3w3) – found in linseeds (flaxseeds), chia seeds, Echium seed, sea buckthorn and walnuts, as well as their oils, the herb purslane, edible algae, mung beans and dark green leafy vegetables, such as kale.

Having optimal amounts of these two have numerous health benefits, including prevention of heart disease and stroke, and reduced joint pain. Deficiencies in LA and ALA lead to many disorders, including depression, suppressed immune function, dryness of skin, reduced growth rates. (Ref. 1)

The essential fatty acid ALA is particularly important for our health as numerous studies suggest that ALA itself reduces inflammation, heart and vascular disease risk, decreases insulin resistance, assists with weight management, and may benefit brain function.

What about omega-3 fatty acids?

Alpha-linolenic acid (ALA) is the parent omega-3 fatty acid from which the body can make the longer chained polyunsaturated omega-3 fatty acids (generally called PUFAs), particularly:

- EPA – eicosapentaenoic acid (20:5w3)
- DHA – docosahexaenoic acid (22:6w3)

As if that is not enough, ALA can also be converted by the body to the less well-known omega-6 gamma-linolenic acid (GLA). You may have seen it labelled on bottles of borage oil (20-24% GLA) and evening primrose oil (8-10% GLA). It is also found in hemp oil and in blackcurrants. GLA is anti-inflammatory and beneficial for reducing symptoms of PMS, arthritis, eczema and psoriasis.

The omega-3s EPA and DHA are not classified as 'essential' i.e. the body can theoretically make them from ALA. However, they are very important for our health and there are two opposing schools of thought as to whether we can actually make sufficient amounts of these or whether we need to get them from our diet (more on this later).

Why are omega-3s so important?

When present in large enough amounts, these polyunsaturated omega-3 fatty acids provide an anti-inflammatory effect on the body. They help to regulate heart rate, blood pressure, blood clotting and fertility. (Ref. 2) They are also needed by the immune system and help to fight infections. They are required for healthy growth of the developing foetus. In children, they are involved in the development of the nervous system. It has even been shown that attention deficit disorder (ADD) is in large part due to the omega-3 fatty acid DHA deficiency (Dr D Amen, University of California). There are receptors in the brain that look for omega-3s, and if they cannot find them, they coagulate causing, the beginnings of dementia and Alzheimer's.

In the early 1980s, my research project, as part of an M.Sc. in Nutrition at London University, involved a double-blind trial. I gave fish oil capsules (containing the two fatty acids, EPA and DHA) to 20 volunteers for one month, and measured the fatty acid content of plasma lipids and platelet function. In those days, fish oils were less well-known and since then, much research has been done on the health benefits of these two fatty acids. My results showed these oils were beneficial in the 20 volunteers, by reducing blood triglycerides (fats) as well as reducing platelets' clotting action, making them less sticky. (Ref. 3)

Where do the fish get their omega-3s from?

Coldwater fish can make EPA and DHA from ALA, but they also get much of their EPA and DHA from eating brown and red marine algae (phytoplankton). These plants are able to make these fatty acids from carbohydrates. (Ref. 4)

If you prefer to avoid eating fish all together, it is possible to find EPA and DHA sourced from sustainably farmed toxin-free plant-based marine algae (phytoplankton). I use Ocean's Alive Marine Phytoplankton.

Omega-3s from fish or plant?

Fish option

There has been a trend in the last few decades to promote the eating of more oily fish for their omega-3 content. There are plenty of experts who believe we are not capable of making omega-3s efficiently enough to be really healthy without eating fish regularly or supplementing with concentrated fish oil.

Geeky science alert

The enzyme Delta-6 desaturase in the human body, that converts ALA, the omega-3s fatty acid from plants, to the longer chained EPA and DHA, becomes impaired as you age. Also, if you are overweight, have high cholesterol, high blood sugar or blood pressure and insulin and leptin resistance, then this enzyme's activity is reduced. Dr Mercola claims that at least 85% of the Western population has therefore impaired conversion using Delta-6 desaturase. This is the main factor, he claims, which points to the need for supplementation with EPA and DHA. Added to this, enzyme cofactors (vitamins B3, B6, C, zinc and magnesium) are essential in optimum amounts for the best working of this enzyme. Mercola concludes that we need high quality omega-3s from fish and sea food.

One study in 2008 with participants, aged 65 or older, showed that eating oily fish at least once per week compared with less than once per week was associated with a halving of the likelihood of developing age-related macular degeneration. (Ref. 5)

The vegetarian argument

Others believe that as long as the diet contains enough of the two essential fatty acids linoleic acid (LA) and linolenic acid (ALA) from vegetarian origin, there is no need to take fish oils. One simple vegetarian way to increase your consumption of omega-3s (ALA) is to eat more linseeds (See Chapter 6, 'Nuts and Seeds'). Walnuts, pumpkin and butternut squash, kidney beans and black beans are also good sources.

Some experts, such as Dr Brian Clement, Director of Hippocrates Health Institute in Florida, say we can get all the omega-3s we need from plant-based fats. (Ref. 6) Clement cynically considers the promotion of fish oils for health to be a decades-old campaign to take people's money and is concerned about the toxicity of fish and fish oils today. He supports the theory that the body can produce EPA and DHA from plant foods and that when you consume them from fish oils, you are reducing the body's ability to make them.

Not only do fish oils contain toxins, as mentioned earlier, but to compound the matter, Clement claims "fish oils [in bottles and capsules] have oxidized...and become rancid, cancer-causing fats." And he says, "EPA and DHA are 25 times more sensitive to the destruction by light, oxygen and heat" than good quality vegetable oils.

One company I have used, called Igennus, makes a high-quality vegetarian omega-3 oil – Echiomega oil from the Echium seed (Vipers Bugloss or Blueweed). They say it "is the richest plant source of the rare omega-3 fatty acid stearidonic acid (SDA). SDA offers an unusually high rate of conversion to the long-chain omega-3s EPA and DHA – up to 5x greater than any other short-chain omega-3, including ALA found in flaxseed oil." Igennus claims that Echium seed oil produces 60% more omega-3 EPA and DHA in the body than linseed oil. (Ref. 7)

Let's look at the advantages and disadvantages of eating whole fish.

Oily fish like herring, sardines and mackerel, also known as forage fish, contain just as many omega-3s as salmon, as well as containing vitamin D and B12. Being lower down the food chain, they tend to harbor far fewer toxins. Experts advise people to consume these smaller fish rather than larger fish, to reduce toxic contamination. According to Alison Barratt of the Monterey Bay Aquarium's Seafood Watch program, forage fish "are theoretically some of the most abundant in the ocean," which is "beneficial if you're looking for fish you can catch in abundance without impacting the population." So fulfilling our seafood needs with forage fish reduces the environmental impact of our diet. (Ref. 8)

In the last 70 years or so, no one can deny that the once cleaner waters of the planet have become horribly polluted, as have the creatures that inhabit them. Tuna may be one of the most polluted fish containing unsafe amounts of mercury, which affects the human nervous system's functioning. Mercury, dioxins and polychlorinated pesticides (PCBs) are commonly found in fish, fish oils and other marine organisms. Even reduced usage of these chemicals by some countries in recent years has not prevented them from remaining in the sea environment and its animals.

Some experts advise to avoid eating fish all together, due to their toxicity, caused mainly by mercury, but more recently by radioactive contamination from Fukushima. One report (Ref. 9) says that 300 tons of radioactive water has been seeping into the Pacific Ocean EVERY DAY since March 15, 2011 and now most marine life in the Pacific Ocean is contaminated, and many animals are dying. Fish caught and tested near the site have tested positive for radioactive particles. Also, bluefin tuna found near California have also tested positive.

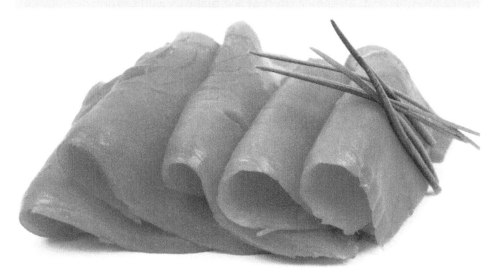

Wild salmon versus farmed salmon

Although wild salmon contains more mercury and now possibly radioactive substances, farmed salmon contains several times higher amounts of chemicals linked with cancer, including pesticides and PCBs, a common environmental pollutant. (Ref. 10 and 11) This is largely due to the feeding of captive fish with ground-up fishmeal that contain accumulated toxins. These fish are further fed toxic dyes to provide a pink shade of colour that the consumer expects. This pink colour, of salmon, prawn and crab's flesh, in nature, is due to the carotenoid, astaxanthin, an antioxidant with many health benefits.

Further disadvantages of farmed salmon are due to the densely-populated metal cages they are kept in, which are known to harbour pesticides, viruses, antibiotics and heavy metals releasing them into the surrounding water. These cages seem cruel to me, as well as causing damage to the seabed. Spread of sea ice is also a problem with tightly packed farmed salmon.

To conclude, it is a difficult choice to make – wild salmon comes with an environmental cost; already a third of the planet's wild salmon population is at risk of extinction. (Ref. 12 and 13) Although Alaska had one of the lowest polluted waters and provided the best source of wild fish, post Fukushima, this may be changing.

What is krill and should we consume krill oil?

Krill are small shrimp-like planktonic crustaceans living in all the oceans of the world. However, the most abundant is Antarctic krill.

From an environmental perspective, the harvesting of krill is debatable. Environmental campaigners say, "The krill population is vital, but it's depleting fast. Research shows krill populations have already dropped by 80 percent since the 1970s," depriving whales and penguins of their food. Not everyone agrees; some say that krill makes up the largest biomass in the world, and its harvesting is regulated by the World Wildlife Fund. They say this harvesting could continue for centuries, making it a highly sustainable source of omega-3s.

From a health perspective, krill oil contains the fatty acids EPA and DHA in a phospholipid form, making them easier to absorb in the gut and meaning that we need far less krill oil per day (1g krill oil versus 3-5g fish oil). And as it contains the light pink astaxanthin, the powerful antioxidant, this keeps the krill oil stable and prevents it from becoming oxidised.

Whether you choose a vegetarian oil, krill oil or a fish oil, I suggest you use the information provided here to make the best choice for you. The quality of the oil is crucial and determined by the manufacturer's efforts to reduce oxidation of the oils during processing and storage. In the case of fish oils, the added factor is choosing the least polluted source.

Balancing Omega-6 with Omega-3 fats

Not only is our body's omega-3 level vital for good health, but the ratio of omega-6s to omega-3s is crucial too. Basically, most people consume 20 times more omega-6s than omega-3s, leading to inflammation and many chronic diseases. Ideally, the ratio of omega-6 to omega-3 should be between 1:1, and no greater than 4:1.

This overconsumption of omega-6s is largely due to the popularity of processed foods (savoury and sweet pastries, cakes, biscuits, crisps and chips) with their high margarine and vegetable oil content (especially corn, sunflower and soybean oils) largely made up of omega-6 fatty acids.

So to address this imbalance, cutting down on omega-6 fatty acids is important, at the same time as supplementing with a high-quality fish oil, a vegetarian oil such as linseed oil, Echiomega capsules, or marine phytoplankton. A family-run linseed farm in Sussex grow, cold press and sell linseed oil that is fresh, as well as whole linseeds (see 'Resources').

If you are interested in investigating your omega-3 levels, you can buy an Opti-O-3 test kit (from Igennus), which measures your red blood cell fatty acid profile. From this test, a report is sent to you recommending what level of omega-3s, you need to take for optimum health. It involves a simple finger prick blood spot onto a card done at home. This can be a useful test to do, for example, when you have been taking the oil of your choice for three months. I found this a good way to measure the effectiveness of the oil I was taking to raise my omega-3s.

Medium Chain Fatty Acids (MCFA)

MCT (medium chain triglyceride) oil is currently a trend, being sold and promoted as a healthy fat, particularly in the athletic and bodybuilding world.

According to Shilhavy (Ref. 14), the MCT oil that is being sold is best avoided as it is processed, containing only tiny amounts of lauric acid, if any. He says it may well be a lucrative way of disposing of coconut oil when the valuable lauric acid has been removed for use in the food, drug and nutraceuticals industry.

MCT oil, used by athletes, is a source of energy for workouts, because MCTs are digested and absorbed more rapidly than other longer chain fatty acids. Also, being smaller, they travel to all parts of the body and are metabolised more rapidly, supplying muscles with fuel. They are also not stored as fat deposits.

Overall, MCT oil's usefulness is limited; it does not supply any EFAs or other nutrients, and can reduce the transport in the blood of useful nutrients like vitamin E, by using up shared carrier proteins. I personally prefer to use coconut oil, as the most natural source of MC fatty acids, (MCFAs).

Geeky science alert

What is MCT? Like any triglyceride, basically it consists of three medium chain fatty acids, all linked to a glycerol molecule.

"Medium" refers to the chain length of the fatty acid, containing between 6 and 12 carbon atoms.

The two most well known MCFAs are Caprylic acid (C8) (highest amounts in goat's milk, butter and cheese) and Lauric acid (C12), which has powerful antimicrobial properties and is the predominant MCFA in coconut oil (approx 50% of its fatty acids). Lauric acid is also found in human breast milk (6-10% lauric acid).

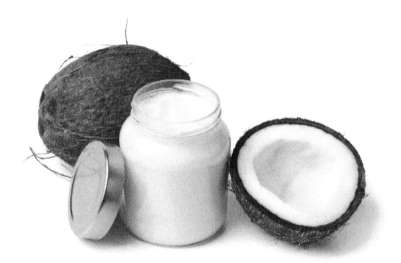

Energy Boosting Tip
from Ann Christiansen, Nia Black Belt teacher trainer
www.anniann.com/en

"My best tip is to start putting butter in my coffee in the morning – and adding some vanilla, cardamom, raw chocolate or some goji berries for taste; it's fun. There's MCT present in good butter – a perfect start. For me, it has changed the way I run my energy each day, and I do very well on it."

Summary

- There are only two fatty acids that are 'essential' to our diet – linoleic acid (LA) and alpha-linolenic (ALA) acid, found in leafy vegetables and nuts/seeds, particularly walnut, sunflower, linseed (freshly ground) and chia.

- ALA may be particularly helpful in reducing inflammation and heart disease, as well as being the parent fatty acid for the beneficial polyunsaturated omega-3 fatty acids, EPA and DHA.

- Omega-3 fatty acids provide an anti-inflammatory effect, as well as lowering plasma triglycerides.

- EPA and DHA are made by marine algae, and the fish incorporate these fatty acids into their fat by eating the algae.

- A vegetarian source of EPA and DHA come from phytoplankton, such as Ocean's Alive Marine Phytoplankton liquid drops.

- Eating oily fish is a source of omega-3s, and may reduce the likelihood of developing macular degeneration.

- Forage fish, like herring and sardines, are lower down the food chain, so accumulate less toxins from the environment than larger fish.

- Consuming forage fish has a lower environmental impact than eating larger fish.

- Overall, eating wild salmon is better for you and the environment than farmed salmon.

- There are vegetarian sources of omega-3s, which some experts believe are better than eating fish or fish oils.

- Although krill oil is a great source of omega-3s, also containing antioxidant astaxanthin, the environmental cost may be too great.

- The ratio of omega-6s to omega-3s should be between 1:1 to 4:1. Aim to keep your consumption of vegetable oil and margarine to a minimum.

- Use a test kit to keep a check on your omega-3 levels.

- Medium chain fatty acids (MCFAs) mostly refer to caprylic and lauric acid. It is best to avoid the MCT oils on the market, which are too synthetic.

- Obtain your MCFAs from small amounts of coconut oil and/or goat's milk, butter or cheese.

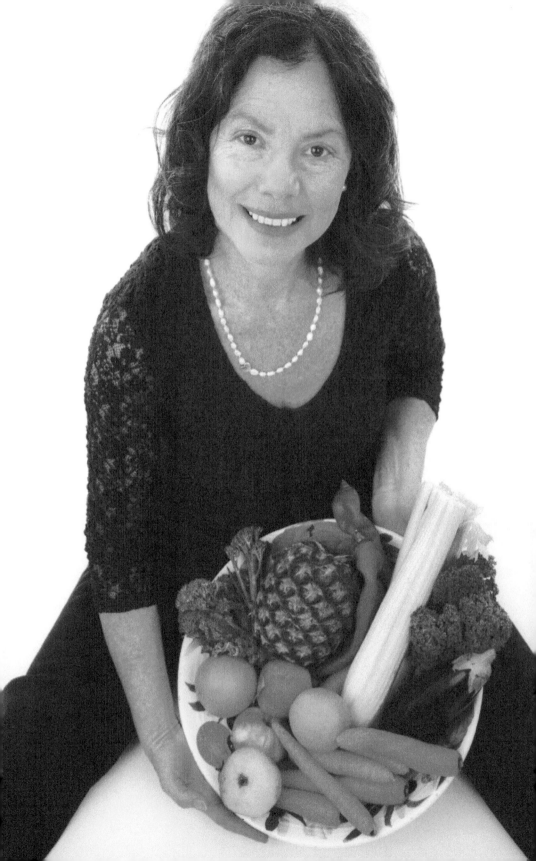

Chapter 8
"To cook or not to cook?"

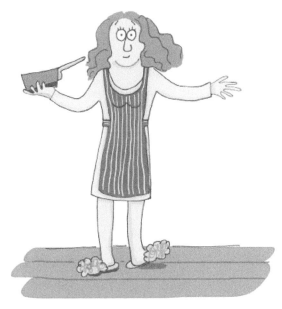

I'm not one of these people that like to spend many hours in the kitchen, so I aim to keep my food preparation simple and as close to nature as possible. However, I do find preparing and cooking food a creative and nurturing act. I love to make simple, tasty and healthy food for my family on a daily basis.

Cooked food is delicious, entertaining, comforting and warming. Heat is also essential for some food, rendering it digestible and safe to eat, such as beans, grains, potatoes and meat. On the other hand, many vegetables and fruit are best eaten raw, so that maximum benefit can be taken from them.

Heat has a large effect on the nutritional value of food. It denatures (destroys) proteins, making them harder to digest, damages fats creating carcinogens, and mainly reduces the amount and availability of nutrients; generally, the hotter and longer you cook food, the more damage is done.

A large percentage of the phytonutrients, including vitamins and many of the minerals, are altered or destroyed, rendering them useless. Viktoras Kulvinskas, in his book *Survival into the 21st Century*, estimates that the overall nutrient destruction is as high as 80%.

The 'Raw food' diet

The 'Raw food' diet has become well-known over the last 20 years, with several celebrities championing it. I am referring to the 'movement', or in some cases 'dogma', that promotes the exclusive eating of uncooked vegan food. There are so many books, websites, and videos to follow on this subject, and I spent a good 10 years researching and experimenting with this type of diet.

As much as I appreciate the value of raw food i.e. juices, smoothies, salads and fruits for nourishing, detoxifying the body and enabling healing to be accelerated, I do not think it is a good idea to exclusively live off raw food on a long-term basis, particularly if you live in Northern climates. My experience has been valuable; as they say, "You live and learn".

Not only did I discover some great new ways to make exciting salads, but also that an all raw meal, day or week (in the summer) is wonderful for detoxifying and increasing vitality. I eat a large salad almost every day, and when I say large, I mean the sort of size most people would think, "That serves four!" I juice at least once a day and make sure I have a smoothie with added ground linseed and green superfood powder (see Chapter 12, 'Superfoods').

As you have read in the previous chapters, raw plants provide thousands of phytonutients, and so it makes sense to include them as a high percentage of your diet, to reduce inflammation and hence aging. I recommend increasing your raw plant intake up to at least 50% in warm summery seasons, as well as all year, if it feels right for your body.

Recipe

This Middle Eastern Salad is always a winner in our household.

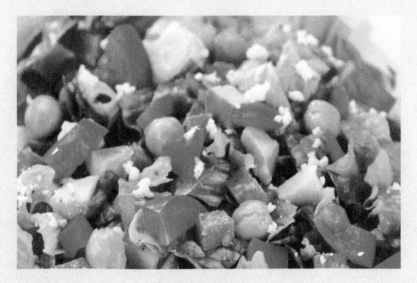

4 ripe tomatoes

1 large cucumber

2 peppers

½ mild onion

1 lemon, juiced

dash of olive oil

fresh herbs, chopped e.g. dill, coriander, parsely

salt (sea salt or Himalayan), to taste

a sprinkling of sumac (optional)

Chop the vegetables into small cubes and mix well.

Dress with lemon and olive oil.

Sprinkle with salt, herbs and sumac.

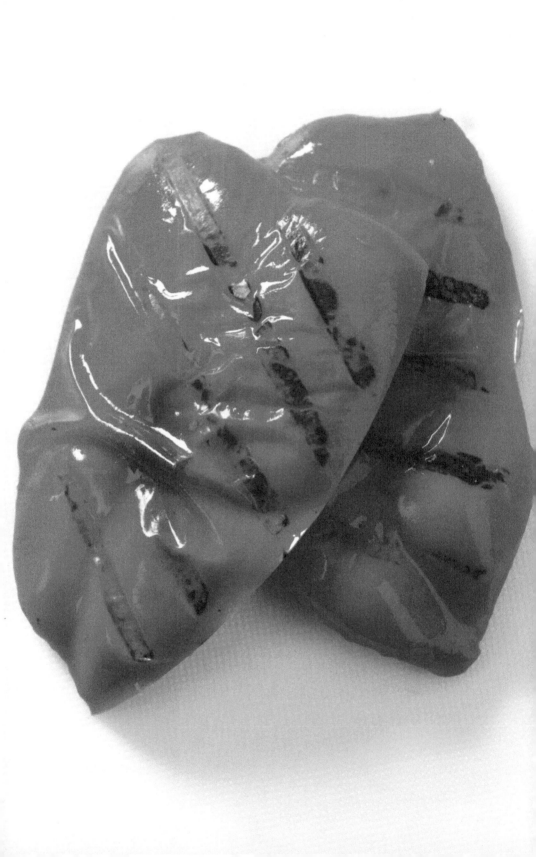

Recipe
Grilled Pepper Salad, or Ardei Copts

My mother loves to cook, and as a young girl, growing up in Romania, learned many local recipes. Here's one of my favourite Romanian childhood dishes, using cooked red and green peppers.

4-6 red and/or green (one pepper per person)
Vinaigrette
3 tbsp olive oil
2 tbsp vinegar (I prefer unpasteurised apple cider vinegar)
sea salt
black pepper

- Place the whole peppers, without cutting off the stalks, directly onto the flames of a gas hob. Traditionally, a charcoal fire was used. It will also work to place peppers under a grill or on a tray in a hot oven.
- Turn the peppers regularly, as the skin cooks and blisters. Keep turning every few minutes until the whole pepper is cooked. Place the cooked pepper in a glass bowl, covering with a lid to keep in the moisture. After about 20 minutes, when cool, they are easy to peel by pulling the skin off. Keep wetting your hands and rubbing the pepper to remove all trace of charred skin. The peppers at this point are whole, although some do fall apart.
- Place in a salad bowl and add a good amount of vinaigrette. This dish is best left to marinate a few hours, or it can be made the day before, but often does not last that long in our house.

The problems with cooked food

If you heat carbohydrates without water e.g. when baking bread or a potato, then acrylamides (which are carcinogenic) form on the crispy surface. If you cook carbohydrates in water, no acrylamides are formed. "What about delicious roast potatoes?" My motto is, "Never say never," so boil your carbohydrates most of the time. It's what you do most of the time that is important. Cooking carbohydrates with water is best as the temperature does not exceed 100ºC.

When foods that contain a mix of sugars, fats, and proteins are cooked, the Maillard reaction occurs. The sugars and proteins in the food react together with heat and form compounds called AGEs (advanced glycation end products). Pasteurisation, drying, smoking, frying, microwaving and grilling can all cause AGE production. They provide flavour, hence not so easy to give up (think toast!)

AGEs contribute to chronic inflammation and aging. Diets with more raw foods typically contain minimal AGEs. Foods with the highest AGEs are meat, butter and processed cream cheese. To avoid AGEs, poach, stew or steam food, and use lower temperatures, moist heat, and don't overcook the food.

Cooking with fats causes further problems. All fats are damaged by heat, but some more than others. Oils are more vulnerable than solid fat as oils contain mono or polyunsaturated fatty acids (more double bonds). This makes them more vulnerable to oxidisation and the forming of harmful free radicals.

Geeky science alert

Free radicals in a nutshell: heat causes the fatty acid molecule to lose an electron and become a 'free radical'. This is what does the damage to DNA and other cell structures, causing aging, and even cancer. How to avoid this damage is to reduce the amount of cooked oils you eat. Second best is to reduce the heat and length of cooking time, and thirdly is to include plenty of antioxidants, such as vitamin C and E, in your diet ... (remember, add plenty of colourful plant foods to your diet). These antioxidants provide the missing electrons and neutralise the free radicals, rendering them harmless.

Many recipes start with, "Chop a small onion and fry in olive oil". Not great if you are attempting to avoid the damaging effects of heated oils and free radicals. A cooking trick that I invented is to 'simmer-fry' a chopped onion in ½ cm of water, and after a minute or so, add some olive oil or coconut oil. The water will ensure that the oil temperature never rises above about 100ºC. You will miss out on the caramelised smell and taste of fried onions, but overall I think it is a small price to pay for good health, and the taste is still great.

Interesting fact

While on the subject of oils,
extra virgin means it is cold pressed,
using pressure to extract the oil from the seed,
without heat or chemical solvents.
Buy extra virgin organic olive oil in
a dark glass bottle for optimum storage.

Grains and gluten

When it comes to grains, it is best to eat the whole grain e.g. brown rice, not white rice. It is less processed, so contains more nutrients and fibre. Likewise, wholemeal flours are better than refined white flour. You may well know how much bread and other wheat products you can tolerate. Many people have a mild (sub-clinical) gluten intolerance, and can tolerate only a small amount of gluten; not to be confused with coeliac disease, which is much more serious and easier to diagnose.

This sub-clinical intolerance may be experienced with symptoms such as bloating, heartburn, constipation, diarrhoea and abdominal pain as well as fatigue, and can go on for years and even decades without you being aware of the hidden wear and tear. Low-grade inflammation of the lining of the small intestinal tract can lower your immune system's strength. It can also result in a condition called leaky gut syndrome, where the lining of the gut lets molecules cross over into the blood stream. These molecules would normally not get through, but be further broken down into smaller molecules by digestion. All of this leakage can lead to allergies with a further weakening of the immune system, blood sugar problems and fatigue.

The predominant grains to avoid if you suspect you do not tolerate gluten are wheat, rye and barley. Increasingly popular are spelt and kamut grains, related to wheat, which some people find they digest well. All these grains contain gluten, but wheat contains the most. The other grains contain less gluten, but still enough to cause inflammation in some people. It's the polypeptide gliadin, found in the gluten protein, that causes the reaction. Avoiding these grains means avoiding bread, pasta, pastries, croissant and many breakfast cereals.

What are the gluten-free alternatives?

Rice, corn, millet, quinoa, amaranth, oats, and buckwheat are generally good (seed) alternatives. Although oats (porridge) does contain a certain amount of gluten, it can usually be well tolerated in sensitive individuals. Once again, it's good to listen to how you feel after eating them. If you do decide to take a break from gluten-containing grains, it can take 30 to 60 days to reduce inflammation in the intestines and up to a year to fully heal the lining of the small intestines.

Energy Boosting Tip
from Ann Christiansen, Nia Black Belt teacher trainer

"No more carbs in the morning keeps my blood sugar level stable, with no cravings, and a good mind focus. No more croissants – ah well. I did eat enough croissants perhaps at a weekend brunch in a niche hotel. I will still eat such things ... but then I know what that will do to the rest of my day."

There are many recipes on the Internet, using the less well-known buckwheat, amaranth and millet. Here's a family favourite recipe modified from the famous Cranks' recipe book:

Recipe
Buckwheat bake

Ingredients:

100g buckwheat

1 medium onion

1 medium carrot

2tbs olive oil

175g red lentils

900ml vegetable stock

2 tbs chopped parsley

a small sprig rosemary, chopped

salt and pepper to taste

nutmeg to taste

- Chop the onion and carrot and simmer-fry in 1cm water for a few minutes.
- Add the buckwheat and lentils and remaining ingredients. Bring to the boil and simmer on low heat for about 30 mins, until the liquid is absorbed.
- Press the mixture into a greased 25cm round flan dish and bake in the oven at 200C or (400F/ Gas mark 6) for 30 mins
- Serve hot or cold with a salad.

Summary

- Cooking is a creative and nurturing activity, creating delicious and comforting dishes.

- Heat destroys and reduces the availability of many nutrients, including proteins, fats, vitamins and minerals.

- Raw foods, such as juices, smoothies and salads as well as fruit, enable the body to be nourished, and can accelerate detoxification and healing.

- Occasional raw food days or weeks can be beneficial, especially in the summer.

- Aim to gradually increase your intake of raw plants to at least 50% of your diet.

- Cooking carbohydrates with water is best. In the absence of water, acrylamide, a carcinogen, is formed.

- AGEs, which cause inflammation and aging, are produced when you heat food containing a mix of sugar and protein.

- Keep cooking with oils and fats to a minimum to avoid production of free radicals, which damage DNA and other cell structures. 'Simmer-fry' instead.

- Eat wholegrains wherever possible.

- Include more non-gluten grains (seeds), such as millet, buckwheat and amaranth, and even exclude all gluten containing grains if you have a problem with them.

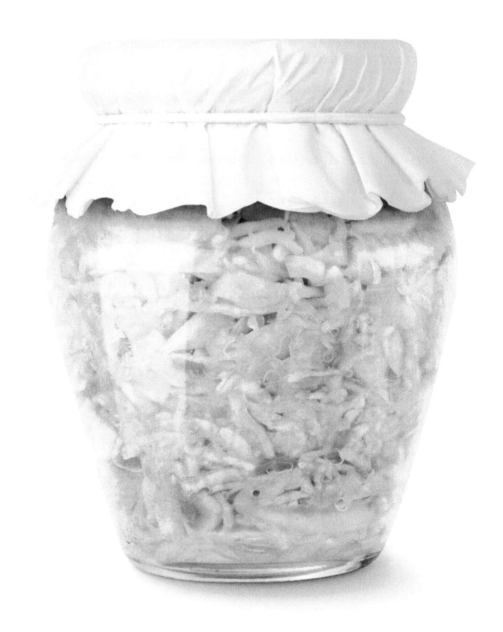

Chapter 9
Fermented Foods and Probiotics

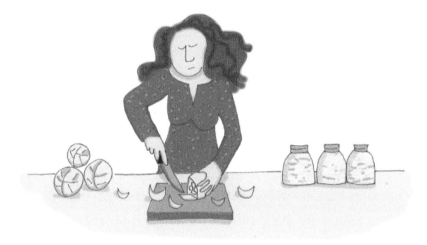

"People in cultures around the world have been eating yogurt, cheeses, and other foods containing live cultures for centuries," says Martin Floch, MD, a professor of gastroenterology at Yale University, co-author of *Probiotics: A Clinical Guide*.

We have 10 times more microbial cells in our body than human cells. That means we are more bacteria, fungi and viruses than human – weird! Our gut is home to trillions of microorganisms, making it an amazing ecosystem, known collectively as the microbiome.

Your microbiome has a profound influence on your health and your immune system. Its make-up varies depending on where you live, what you eat and your health history.

One of the best ways of protecting your health is by keeping your gut microflora healthy. There is a lot we still don't know about our microbiome, but we do know that the genes of our microbes send signals to our brain, helping with food cravings, as well as communicating directly with our immune system.

Your gut health and immune system are closely linked with approximately 70 to 80% of your immune tissue, located within your digestive system. The gut is often the first entry point for exposure to pathogens (bad bacteria and viruses that can cause disease); therefore, your gut immune system needs to be thriving and healthy in order to avoid illness.

All the more reason to avoid antibiotics, if at all possible, and food contaminated with antibiotics, such as non-organic meat and milk, which may harm the vital gut ecosystem.

Eating fermented foods daily is the cheapest way to ensure you are getting a good probiotic. Eat a small amount (2-3 tbsp) of sauerkraut or other fermented vegetables with each meal (see the following recipe). Raw miso or fermented organic dairy (yoghurt) are good alternatives. Many commercial yoghurts can contain artificial preservatives, sweeteners such as high fructose corn syrup (HFCS), even titanium dioxide! And they don't necessarily contain very many beneficial bacteria.

Another way to look after and maintain a healthy microbiome is to take a high-quality probiotic. Make sure you find one that provides about 20 to 30 billion live bacteria per capsule.

Sauerkraut – the Ultimate Superfood

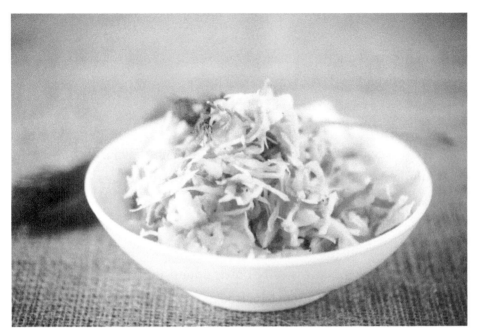

Raw sauerkraut is easy to make and when fresh, organic and raw (unlike most jars found in the shops), digestion is greatly enhanced. It also helps to re-establish and maintain a healthy inner ecosystem.

The benefits of sauerkraut are:

- very easy to digest, having been predigested by the friendly bacteria

- will aid in the digestion of any foods eaten at the same meal

- helps with digestive problems

- rich in 'live' beneficial bacteria (lactobacilli) and vitamin K2

- good for appetite control and sugar cravings

Sauerkraut recipe

Here's my tried and tested sauerkraut recipe. I can't tell you how many foul-smelling jars of sauerkraut landed on my compost heap before I discovered and modified this recipe.

- Choose a firm white or green cabbage (my favourite one is the light-green sweetheart cabbage, as it produces the best sauerkraut).

- Chop the cabbage in half to remove the core, then finely chop the two halves. In a sturdy bowl, pound the cabbage with a rolling pin end, or other similar kitchen tool, for 10 minutes. Then sprinkle with 1 tsp sea salt or Himalayan salt, and cover with cloth or plate. Leave overnight.

- The following morning, take a Kilner or Mason jar, and fill the jar with about 2 cm of the chopped cabbage. Push and gently pound it down, using the rolling pin again. Keep repeating this until the jar is nearly full. The pounding down is very important to exclude air.

- Make a brine solution: 1 tsp sea salt/Himalayan salt with 250ml boiled cool water.

- Optional: Add 1 capsule of probiotic (cracked open) to the solution and mix. Pour this solution over the cabbage until it is submerged. Use a crock or weight to keep the cabbage submerged at all times.

- Leave at room temperature. It will take anything from three days to a week to ferment. When it tastes tangy, it is ready. Store it in the fridge or in cool conditions to slow down the fermentation. Remember, it's alive! Enjoy.

NB: You can also layer other vegetables, such as chopped up chard, kale or carrots, and also spices e.g. juniper berries or caraway seeds.

Summary

- Looking after your gut microorganisms may increase the health of your immune system.

- Avoid antibiotics, if at all possible, and food that contains antibiotics.

- Eating fermented food daily is a good way to take a probiotic e.g. sauerkraut, live yoghurt.

- Or take a high-quality probiotic capsule.

- Make your own sauerkraut with this simple recipe.

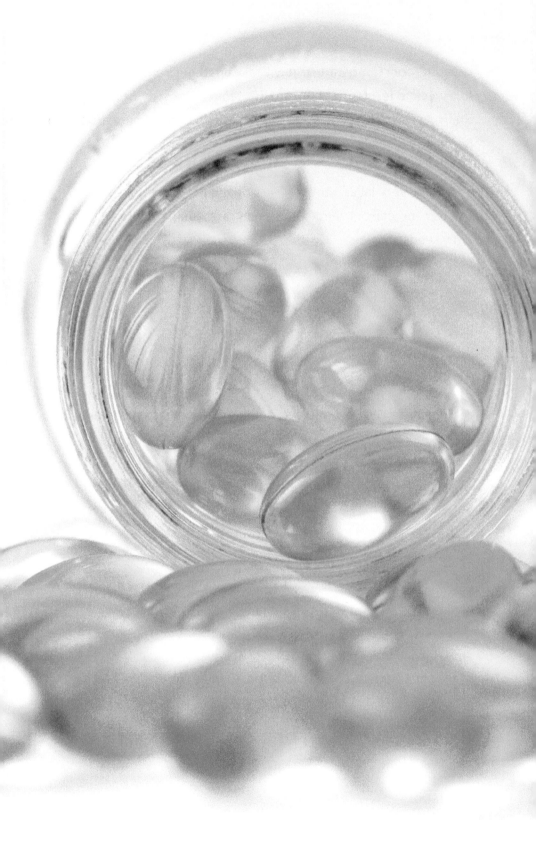

Chapter 10

Supplements

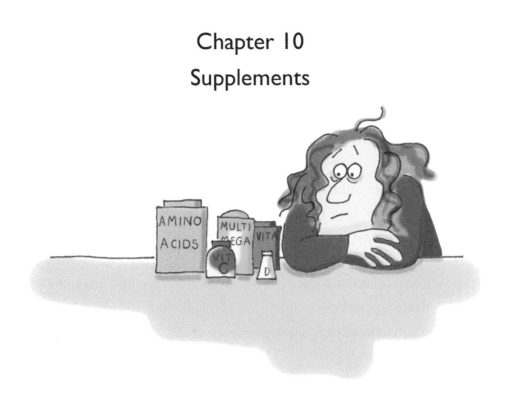

Supplements are by no means an alternative to a wholesome plant-based diet, but possibly a valuable addition, at certain times, to enable you to feel fabulous and function optimally.

I can almost hear you say, "Oh, I really don't want to take loads of pills and capsules every day, and the cost adds up."

Some say the cost and hassle of remembering to take supplements is worth it, better than having to take prescribed medication now or at any time in the future, for an illness you could have prevented! Others say a healthy diet and superfoods is the way to go. More on superfoods in Chapter 12. Yet again, only you can use your intuition to decide what feels right and makes you feel well.

To supplement or not?

When Hippocrates said, "Let thy food be thy medicine and thy medicine be thy food," he was describing nature's promise to provide us with good health and a long life, through the eating of whole foods. This did not include the introduction of a myriad of synthetic nutrients that have become widely available, centuries later, nor the 'fortification' or 'enrichment' of certain foods, such as flour, with synthetic nutrients, that 'guinea pig' humans all over the world are unwittingly consuming.

Vitamins and minerals are classified as 'essential' in our diet, meaning the body is unable to synthesise them, and they must be absorbed from the diet, be it from whole foods or supplements.

There are thousands, if not millions, of natural molecules in food (many we have yet to identify) which work synergistically with each other. Let's take beta-carotene, the vitamin A precursor, the yellow/orange antioxidant seen in carrots and tomatoes, that the body converts to Vitamin A.

It always occurs naturally together with other antioxidants, such as alpha and gamma carotene, as these all require each other for their synergistic roles. So the eating of whole, organic, unprocessed foods is the ideal to strive for. Isolated nutrients are no substitute for pure foods in their ability to promote and maintain health. Yet from many different sources, we are led to believe we need to supplement what we eat, that food alone is no longer sufficient to maintain health and prevent chronic diseases.

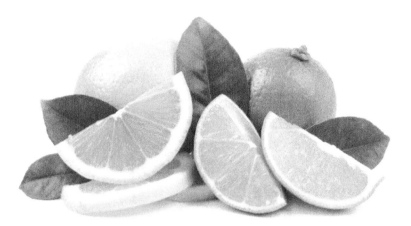

As long ago as the 1700s, Lind found that lemons and limes prevented sailors getting scurvy, due to their vitamin C content. He had 'supplemented' the sailors using the juice from the whole fruit. More recently, over the last 40 or so years, a huge number of studies have shown that supplements do have a range of health benefits e.g. chromium can reduce depression as well as improve blood sugar control in diabetes.

There is so much evidence now that diet alone, even a good one, cannot provide all the vitamins and minerals that we need. Why is this? Nutrient levels in plant foods have generally declined during the twentieth century, largely because of the reduction in quality of the soil across the whole planet due to the use of synthetic fertilisers, pesticides and herbicides. Measurements in the US between 1973 and 1997 showed calcium levels in broccoli dropped by 53%, vitamin B1 by 35% and niacin by 29%. (Ref. 1) I strongly believe that we need to make organic and biodynamic farming principles, as well as permaculture, a priority with the aim to improve and restore the correct mineral balance and overall health of the soil. Eventually, this will improve and restore the nutrient content of plant food, but there is a long way to go and it will take time.

Each of us can contribute to this with our own organic vegetable patches and pots, even adding vegetables to our flower beds. See 'Incredible Edible' and 'Guerrilla Gardening' in 'Resources' for inspiration.

Another factor in nutrient decline is that the food we buy is rarely 'freshly picked', resulting in a reduction in vitamins and other nutrients. The processing of food, sometimes to high temperatures, and the addition of preservatives and other additives, further reduces the nutrients that are available for absorption. Added to this the increased stresses of modern life as well as the increased level of toxic pollutants in our bodies may increase our vitamin and mineral requirements.

Meanwhile, most people are not even consuming large enough amounts of vegetables daily to maintain good health, let alone protect against chronic disease.

To summarise:

- on the one hand, experts say that the only way to guarantee getting optimum nutrients is through supplementation, ideally with naturally occurring, non-synthetic vitamins and minerals

- but on the other hand, some experts say that all supplements get washed through, doing very little good and end up producing expensive urine,

Ultimately, you will decide whether you can rely solely on your diet for all your nutrients, or whether you will add isolated nutrients, such as vitamins and minerals. You can also decide whether you do this for short periods of time, when you are in need of extra help in healing, or whether you take supplements on a long-term basis. I have learned not to be dogmatic about any of this, to remain flexible enough to change my mind.

Just like life, situations change, and so too does your body as it moves through different stages. Learning to listen to your body as a guide is the best way to navigate this journey of living well and aging well, naturally. Try the body sway test with a supplement to see if it is right for you at this time. Another option is to take advice from a natural health practitioner that you feel aligned with.

Natural supplements versus synthetic ones

Not all supplements are similar in quality. It may surprise you, even shock you, to realise that synthetic vitamins make up the majority of vitamins sold throughout the world today, made by companies that are owned or controlled by pharmaceutical companies; and at least 95% of all vitamin supplements contain some synthetic ingredients, according to Brian R. Clement in his book, *Supplements Exposed*.

The word 'natural' on supplement bottles has been used and abused for so long that there is now no guarantee that the contents are free from synthetic compounds. By law, a vitamin need only contain 10% natural plant derived ingredients to be called natural. Likewise, label claims of 'food source' supplements are misleading, as it only requires that the base is derived from natural 'food' such as yeast, while the addition of synthetic nutrients can be added. However, supplements labelled 'Whole Food' are more likely to be natural and free of synthetic ingredients and, as the name suggests, made from a concentrated whole food.

How natural supplements are made

To make a natural B1 vitamin supplement, often wheat or rice germ is taken as the base food, and mixed with purified water. The fibre is then removed to increase the vitamin's absorption. Dried at low temperatures, it is then tested and made into capsules, using vegetarian gel, ideally without artificial binders, and fillers, such as magnesium stearate.

How synthetic supplements are made

In contrast, synthetic supplements are created entirely through chemistry, often from petrochemicals. If we look at synthetic vitamin B1, often coal tar, derived from fossil fuel, is the base material. Coal tar is widely used not only in the synthesis of vitamins, but also in the food and cosmetics industry, and at certain concentrations can be carcinogenic. Added to it is hydrochloric acid, and after several steps involving heating, cooling, drying and testing, the final synthetic vitamin is sold to distributors and manufacturers. Tablets are formed with the addition of binders and fillers, some of which are toxic. Capsules can be made from gelatin taken from beef and pork hide. Others use the more desirable vegetable sources e.g. cellulose.

Early tests with isolated and synthetic vitamins were useful, but led to an erroneous belief that vitamins were as effective in their isolated state as in their natural whole food state. Vitamins can only function in the presence of their numerous cofactors (which are sometimes minerals). Where vitamins occur in their natural state, these cofactors are present, and the vitamin functions optimally, but in an isolated and synthetic form, not only is its function reduced (Ref. 2), but it can weaken the immune system and even become toxic to the body. Synthetic vitamins and pharmaceutical grade supplements, like drugs, can initially seem to be beneficial, but in time they too can produce harmful side effects and be toxic.

The body cannot be tricked. Chemically derived vitamins are less biologically active, but the manufacturers want you to think that they are the same in their effectiveness, because the synthetic ones are more profitable.

Additives to watch out for!

Look out for what is added to supplements too. There are fillers, binders, lubricants, disintegrants, flavourings and colouring agents, coating materials, and preservatives. Dr Zoltan Rona, medical editor of *The Encyclopedia of Natural Healing*, says that these additives are not toxic to healthy individuals in small amounts, but their consumption over a long period of time may be dangerous. Look out for any of these additives listed on bottle labels, and avoid them.

Common fillers:

- talc (a known carcinogen)
- silicon, which may cause digestion and absorption problems

Artificial colourings (extracted from coal tar), especially the red variety, Red 40 Lake, are carcinogenic.

Synthetic flavourings and sweeteners may be extremely harmful, as they fuel viruses, bacteria and cancers.

Flow agents:

- silicon dioxide known to cause hardening of the arteries
- magnesium stearate, which is often made with hydrogenated fats, making it toxic

Soft gel vitamins often have partially hydrogentated soya bean oil added as a filler, the very same oil linked to causing stroke and heart disease.

Emulsifier and binder
- polyethylene glycol 3350, a hormone disruptor and toxic.

Whitening agent
- titanium dioxide, which may cause pulmonary irritation

For a fuller list and explanation, see Ref. 1, Brian R Clement's book *Supplements Exposed*.

How to find natural supplements
Find products labeled with the words 'whole foods'. Look out for products where care has been taken in the growing, harvesting and preserving of the product, without damage to the environment.

Personally, I like to take a few carefully chosen natural supplements, some superfoods, and the best diet I can ongoingly create!

For my vitamin C supplement, I like to take camu camu, a dried and powdered fruit, which apparently contains more vitamin C that any other food, as it is a 'whole food'! For my multivitamin input, the best one for me is a daily glass of fresh vegetable juice!

Summary

- Supplements may be a valuable addition to a healthy diet at certain times of your life, not necessarily always.

- The toxic environment that we live in increases our requirement for certain nutrients.

- Nutrient levels in plant foods has declined during the last 100 years or so due to artificial farming practices, as well as produce storage time increasing and food processing.

- The ideal to strive for is whole, organic, unprocessed food containing many nutrients, that all work synergistically with each other.

- Ultimately, choose a natural supplement, decide what is right for your body and your situation by listening to how you feel. Or consult a natural health practitioner.

- Synthetic supplements, often made from petrochemicals, may become toxic, be less effective over time, and produce side effects.

- Avoid products containing the listed additives.

- Find 'whole food' supplements that are made by a company that promote care when growing and producing the supplement.

Chapter 11
Vitamin D and Cancer prevention

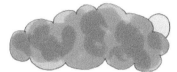

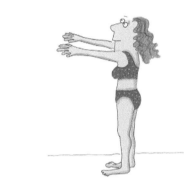

Although vitamin D is indeed a supplement, I feel that it deserves a chapter all of its own. Over the last decade, it has become apparent through countless studies that vitamin D is way more important than 'merely' keeping our bones and teeth healthy.

It is common knowledge that our skin is capable of making vitamin D when exposed to sunlight. However, what we don't realise is that most of us are not in the sun for long enough, with enough of our skin exposed to provide enough vitamin D for optimum health and disease prevention.

Only UVB solar radiation makes vitamin D in our skin, not UVA, and the amount of UVB present depends on the angle of the sun's rays and latitude i.e. how far you are from the equator. In the UK, we are at a latitude of 50-58. Rome and New York are a bit better with 41, but none of these locations have sufficient UVB sunlight, so it's not good news when compared to Bali, with a latitude of 8.

Food sources

Oily fish, milk and eggs provide some vitamin D, but you would need to eat ridiculously large amounts to provide your body with the new higher daily recommendations (see below). For example, eggs are often listed as a good source. In reality, one egg contains 20 IU, so you would need to eat a lot of eggs in one day to make it up to the original RDA (Recommended Daily Amount) of 400 IU, never mind the massively higher new levels of 1-5,000 IU that experts are recommending. Some yoghurts are fortified with Vitamin D, but this does not mean the yoghurt meets other nutritional standards, with respect to sugar and additives.

The long and short of it is that we need to supplement. (Ref. 1) Vitamin D can be taken as an oral spray, or as a capsule. (See 'Resources')

Why supplement?

There may be many potentially therapeutic benefits of Vitamin D supplementation, such as:

- helping to prevent many different types of cancer and slow down the production of cancer cells
- reduce the risk of other conditions, including Type 2 diabetes
- reduce the risk of age-related macular degeneration
- slow the development of Alzheimer's disease
- generally improve infection-fighting abilities.

Carole Braggley is Director of GrassrootsHealth, a public Health Promotion Organisation whose mission it is to increase awareness about vitamin D worldwide, and the crucial role it plays in many aspects of your health.

Vitamin D has powerful effects when it comes to breast cancer, to the degree that breast cancer is being described by some as a "vitamin D deficiency syndrome."

All too often, I've heard women (friends and clients) say, "I thought I was well until I discovered I had breast cancer". This means people often actually feel OK. It appears there are few warning signs or we are too asleep to notice them. Emotional and physiological stress builds in a person over years, and sometimes an emotional crisis can precipitate the body, which is already functioning suboptimally, into a cancer situation. In 2012, nearly 1.7 million new cases of breast cancer were diagnosed worldwide, accounting for 25% of all new cancer cases in women. (Ref. 2)

What can we do about this dire modern cancer predicament?

Carole believes that 90% of ordinary breast cancer is related to vitamin D deficiency – which is 100% preventable! And a study in the journal *Anticancer* (Ref. 3) in 2014 found that higher Vitamin D levels (serum 25(OH)D concentrations) were associated with lower fatality rates in patients with breast cancer. Patients with the highest concentration of vitamin D had approximately half the fatality rate compared to those with the lowest concentration.

Every year, with more research, vitamin D's critical importance seems to be growing. Some say Vitamin D is actually a fat-soluble hormone, made by the body. There are many forms of Vitamin D; the two most important ones are Vitamin D-2 and vitamin D-3 (cholecalciferol). It is D-3, cholecalciferol, that is made naturally by your skin in sunlight.

How much vitamin D do you need to take?

According to John Jacob Cannell, M.D., executive director of the US-based Vitamin D Council, there is no easy answer, as it varies with "age, body weight, percent of body fat, latitude, skin colouration, season of the year, use of sunblock, individual variation in sun exposure, and – probably – how ill you are. Cannell adds, "Vitamin D is used by the body – metabolically cleared – both to maintain wellness and to treat disease. If you get an infection, how much vitamin D does your body use up fighting the infection? If you have cancer, how much vitamin D does your body use up fighting the cancer? Nobody knows the answer to these questions."

Cannell gives the following supplementation guidelines for those who have little UVB exposure: "1,000 IU per every 25 pounds of body weight per day. Healthy adults and adolescents should take 5,000 IU per day. Around 2–3 months later, have a blood test."

The RDA for vitamin D in UK is 400 IU, but many experts believe that while this is enough to prevent the vitamin D deficiency disease rickets, it is way below the amount needed to provide optimum health. On the other hand, a dose of 5,000 IU a day is regarded by many to be safe. At the same time, many practitioners recommend having your blood tested every few months if you are taking high doses like this, as we all metabolise it differently, and in rare cases an excess of it can build up and cause problems.

It's a good idea to get your vitamin D tested using the reliable 25(OH)D test, and supplement as necessary to maintain blood levels in the ideal range.

One particularly noteworthy study was completed by Joan Lappe and Robert Heaney in 2007, (Ref. 4) in which a group of menopausal women were given enough vitamin D to raise their serum levels to 40 ng/ml.

These women experienced a 77% reduction in the incidence of all cancers, across the board, after just four years. (GrassrootsHealth)

As already discussed, a serum Vitamin D of 40 ng/ml is a relatively modest level. The latest information suggests an optimum serum level is 50 to 70 ng/ml. To have such stunning findings in the above study, at just 40 ng/ml supplementation underlines just how powerful and important vitamin D is to your body's optimal functioning.

Vitamin K2's delicate dance with Vitamin D

Vitamin K2 engages in a delicate dance with vitamin D, and you need both in adequate amounts for optimal health. If you take supplemental vitamin D, you also need to make sure you're getting enough vitamin K2. One of vitamin D's roles is to provide improved bone development by helping you absorb calcium. But there is new evidence that vitamin K2 directs the calcium to your skeleton, while preventing it from being deposited where you don't want it, for example, in your organs, joint spaces and arteries. A large part of arterial plaque consists of calcium deposits (atherosclerosis), hence the term "hardening of the arteries".

Sources of vitamin K2

Fermented vegetables can be a great source of vitamin K2 (see Chapter 9, Sauerkraut recipe). Gouda, Brie and Edam cheese are also good sources of vitamin K2.

Whether the body can make vitamin K2 from K1 is debatable. Dr Cannell believes the body can make vitamin K2 from K1. He presents several studies to show this. He concludes, "... as far as getting enough vitamin K2, the best thing to do is eat your greens", which are rich in vitamin K1 (Ref. 5)

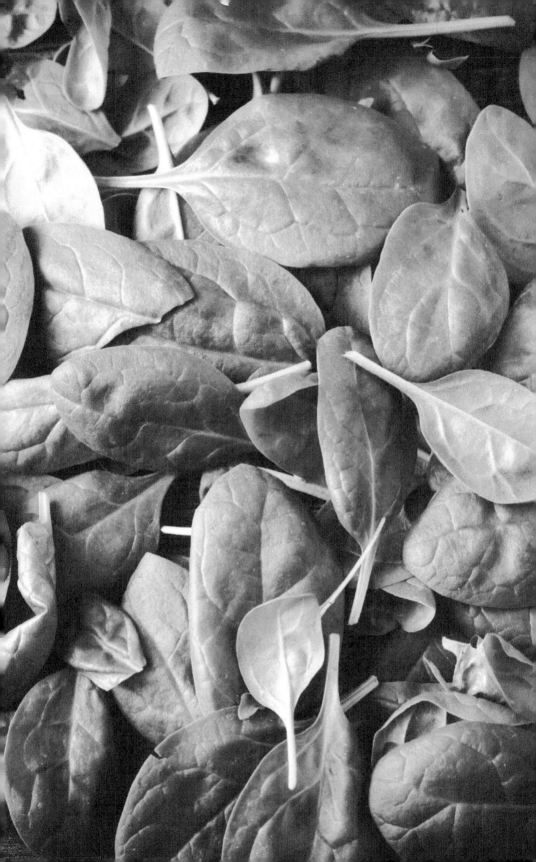

Some good sources of vitamin K1 are: spinach, swiss chard, turnip greens, mustard greens, Brussel sprouts, parsley, romaine lettuce, broccoli, asparagus, collard greens, celery, green beans, leeks, cabbage, basil, thyme, sage and kale. Another option is to take a vitamin K2 supplement. Mercola suggests 150 mcg/day (Ref. 6)

My story on Vitamin D

In 2009, I found Carole Braggley's Grassroots website (see 'Resources') and decided to sign up and be part of a long-term epidemiological study on Vitamin D. This involves paying approx $50/year and twice yearly having my level of vitamin D tested. So every six months, I receive a vitamin D test kit from the USA. All that's involved is placing a blood spot onto a test card and returning it along with completing an online health and fitness questionnaire. My vitamin D results are emailed back to me approximately three weeks later.

My first test results were alarmingly in the red zone – 13 ng/ml serum level of 25(OH)vitamin D. Using the chart provided on the GrassrootsHealth website, I determined how much vitamin D I needed to take daily to raise my levels. Using an oral Vitamin D spray and later a capsule, I took 9,000 IU/day and later reduced it to 6,000 IU/day. Within six months, my levels more than doubled. Five years later, I am happy to say my level of vitamin D3 is 50 ng/ml, which is within the optimum range.

Finally, when getting your Vitamin D levels tested by your doctor, be sure to request the 25(OH)D test specifically (a much more reliable test than the 1,25-dihydroxy-vitamin D test that some doctors will order).

NB: UK serum levels of Vitamin D3 are measured in different units to the USA. On the Grassroots website, there is a converter which makes it easy to compare like with like e.g. 50 ng/ml in USA is the same as 124.8 nmol/litre in UK.

Summary

- Vitamin D plays a role in not only keeping our bones and teeth healthy, but also may be involved in reducing the risk of many cancers, and other diseases too.

- Some describe breast cancer as a vitamin D deficiency syndrome. High serum vitamin D levels have been associated with lower fatality rates in breast cancer patients.

- Although we make vitamin D in the skin when exposed to sunlight, the amount is dependent on latitude, for sufficient UVB rays.

- Most adults should take 1,000-5,000IU/day and have their serum levels of 25(OH)D tested every three months.

- It is important to also take vitamin K2 if you are taking vitamin D, as vitamin K2 directs the calcium to bones rather than depositing it in other tissue, such as the arteries.

- Vitamin K2 is present in some fermented foods, as well as some cheeses, and may be made from vitamin K1 (found in many green and leafy vegetables).

Chapter 12
Superfoods

The relatively new term 'Superfood' is now widely used to describe both some common foods (e.g. blueberries and blackberries) and some less common ones (e.g. goji berries, spirulina). Superfoods offer the most natural, complete and raw form of nutrients available. They contain a high concentration of nutrients and phytochemicals that are shown to have health benefits beyond those of 'common' foods. Yet they do not, on their own, when consumed, cure any disease, nor do they create health miracles, if a poor diet and lifestyle is not addressed.

Superfoods can successfully be added to a current healthy diet to increase the nutrient value of the diet. The superfoods that I like to consume, apart from the berries and green salad leaves I have already mentioned earlier, are:

- turmeric and its active ingredient, curcumin – antioxidant properties
- ginger – sooths digestive system
- Camu camu – for vitamin C
- Spirulina – contains many nutrients
- Chlorella – edible green algae that helps the body to detoxify
- Green powder mixture – high in minerals, containing a blend of dried leaves, barley grass, wheatgrass and marine plants e.g. kelp and blue-green algae

Turmeric – root and powder

You and I know turmeric as that wonderfully vibrant orange-yellow powder we add to curries. Turmeric (Curcuma longa) is an indigenous plant of Asia with a 6,000-year track record as a powerful, yet safe herb in Ayurvedic medicine and Traditional Chinese medicine.

A cousin to ginger, it is also the root of the turmeric, not the broad green leaves, that we are interested in. There has been a relatively recent explosion of interest in its use for promoting and protecting health. It has almost become a superfood superstar!

Juice it!

The whole turmeric root is available from some health food stores and is valuable for juicing. Here's what I do with it:

Juice 1-2 cm turmeric root along with carrots, ginger and whole lemon plus a dash of olive oil (for optimum absorption of the fat-soluble curcumin).

Hundreds of health benefits have been discovered and documented using whole turmeric, as well as the extracted active component, curcumin. There appears to be no toxicity, making it safe to take over time. This key compound, the polyphenol, curcumin, is responsible for most of its medicinal properties and gives the orange colour to turmeric.

Although some say that the turmeric root only contains 1% curcumin, which is hard for the body to absorb, there is always value, in my view, in taking the whole food, with all its other naturally occurring synergistic nutrients. So there is a place for taking turmeric as well as the extracted active ingredient curcumin.

Dr William LaValley, a leading natural medicine cancer physician, has spent much time looking at curcumin's anticancer activity. Curcumin seems to be effective with a wide range of different cancers and has the ability to both destroy cancer cells and promote healthy cell function. It also promotes anti-angiogenesis (helps prevent the development of additional blood supply necessary for cancer cell growth), and affects more than 100 different molecular pathways once it gets into a cell. (Ref. 1)

Another study published in the *Indian Journal of Medical Research* compared the effect of taking oral curcumin with two powerful anti-inflammatory medications, cortisol and phenylbutazone. The study found that curcumin was just as effective in reducing inflammation.

A study in 2011 gave patients with osteoarthritis 200mg curcumin per day, as well as their regular treatment plan, and they had reduced pain and increased mobility (Ref. 2)

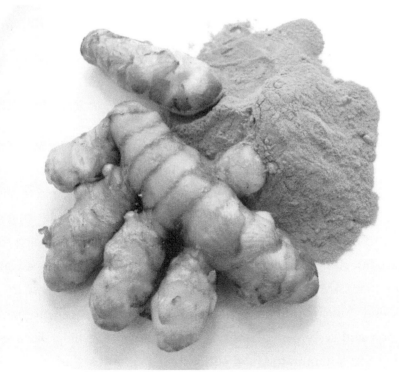

Here's a summary of the health effects of taking curcumin:

- It has been called the number one anticancer spice and defends against breast cancer in many ways. One powerful way it helps reduce the risk of cancer is by helping the liver to break down toxins and prevent carcinogens from forming.

- As an antioxidant, it helps to reduce and neutralise free radicals, which damage and destroy your cells and their DNA. Curcumin also reduces two inflammation-promoting enzymes in your body, and is therefore an effective anti-inflammatory agent.

- It may help inhibit the build up of destructive beta-amyloids in the brain of Alzheimer's patients, as well as break up existing plaques.

- Curcumin has been shown to stabilise blood sugar and reverse cellular insulin resistance by increasing the number of insulin receptors and improving the receptor binding capacity to insulin. (Ref. 3)

Geeky science alert

A research team from Oregon State University has released the result of a study in the *Journal of Nutritional Biochemistry* that demonstrates how curcumin exerts a measurable increase in levels of a protein, cathelicidin antimicrobial peptide, or CAMP, that's known to be important in the "innate" immune system, helping to prevent infection in humans and other animals. Prior to this, it was known that CAMP levels were increased by vitamin D. New research has found that curcumin and vitamin D work synergistically to fight infection and systemic inflammation, as they both exhibit disease-fighting anti-inflammatory and antioxidant properties. (Ref. 4)

Turmeric is the fourth highest antioxidant-rich herb, with an extraordinarily impressive ORAC (Oxygen Radical Absorbance Capacity) score of 159,277. Turmeric also boosts levels of natural cellular antioxidants, such as glutathione, superoxide dismutase, and catalase. These molecules are critical for the body to limit oxidative stress all day long. The greater the surplus of cellular antioxidants, the less stress and damage occurs to vital organ systems.

How to take turmeric or curcumin?

For preventative measures, add turmeric, daily, to your cooked vegetable dishes, to your juices or smoothies. Taking it with some form of healthy fat may improve its absorption. Dr Christine Horner, author of *Waking the Warrior Goddess - Dr Christine Horner's Program to Protect Against & Fight Breast Cancer*, says it's best to add turmeric to your dish near the end of cooking, as it's healing properties are most powerful if it is lightly cooked. A quarter of a teaspoon should be added for each serving.

A therapeutic dose for supporting the body to heal from a serious health condition would be 1,500-1800mg daily of curcumin. "According to Dr LaValley, typical anticancer doses are up to three grams of good bioavailable curcumin extract, three to four times daily." (Ref. 5)

However, as part of your anti-aging plan, consider taking 750mg curcumin in capsule form.

CAMU-CAMU

Myrciaria dubia

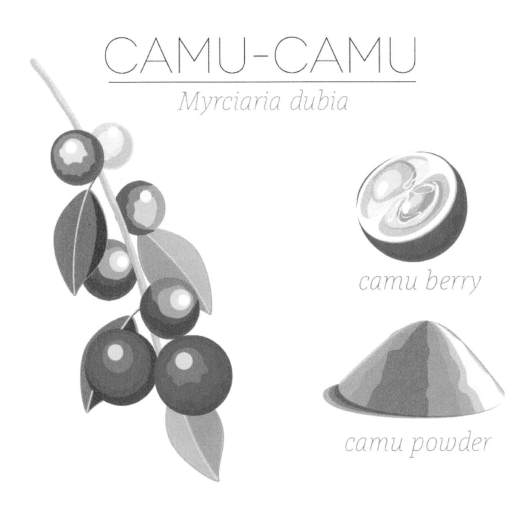

camu berry

camu powder

Ginger

This root has a long history of use for relieving digestive problems, such as nausea, loss of appetite, motion sickness and pain.

It is also associated with reducing pain and inflammation. It does contain numerous anti-inflammatory and antioxidant compounds, such as gingerols, beta-carotene, capsaicin, caffeic acid, curcumin and salicylate.

How to add more ginger to your life:

- Add a 1-2cm piece of fresh ginger to your next smoothie or juice.
- Add fresh, grated or dried ginger to your next stir-fry or home-made salad dressing.
- Add a few thin slices of fresh ginger to a cup of hot water. I love to add slices to my green tea.

Camu camu

Camu camu is a low-growing shrub that grows in the Amazon rainforests of Peru and Brazil. It produces a lemon-sized, light-orange to purplish-red fruit. When dried and made into a powder, it is a potent form of vitamin C.

This powder contains more Vitamin C than any other food, being about 15% Vitamin C by weight! In comparison to oranges, camu camu provides thirty to fifty times more vitamin C, ten times more iron, three times more niacin, twice as much riboflavin, and fifty percent more phosphorus. It is a powerful antioxidant, is antiviral and generally strengthens the immune system. It also helps reduce inflammation and protects the liver.

Being a whole food, I really like this form of vitamin C, knowing it will contain all the synergistic cofactors needed for vitamin C to function well. And it contains NO synthetic additives.

Spirulina

Spirulina is often referred to as a blue-green algae, but it is actually a bacteria that is capable of using the sun to photosynthesise and so obtain its energy. Some people say that, gram for gram, it is the most nutritious food on the planet, with its protein quality being excellent. It is extremely high in many other nutrients too (B vitamins, copper and iron).

Studies have shown that spirulina can help to lower chronic inflammation, has anticancer properties, reduce blood pressure, and even protects against anaemia.

You can take it in tablet form or 1-2 tsp of the powdered form, mixed in with your juice or smoothie.

Chlorella

Chlorella is an edible green algae that grows in fresh water. It is a good source of protein, fats, carbohydrates, fibre, chlorophyll, vitamins, and minerals, BUT the cell wall of chlorella must be broken down before people can benefit from its contents. So when buying chlorella, make sure you are getting "broken cell" chlorella. I take chlorella most days, either as an ingredient in a green superfood powder mix (there are many to choose from on the market), or as chlorella tablets, along with my juice.

Chlorella supports the body's ability to deal with the everyday demands and cope better with our polluted environment. (See Chapter 7, 'Fatty Fishy Facts') Chlorella may help by lowering blood cholesterol and triglycerides, improving the function of your liver, and strengthening your cardiovascular system.

Chlorella also stimulates the growth of friendly gut bacteria, which has the effect of strengthening your microbiome, intestinal microflora, in order to improve your digestion. It may help to treat ulcers, colitis, Crohn's disease, and diverticulosis.

Finally, chlorella may:

- stimulate the immune system, increasing white blood cell counts, preventing colds
- reduce radiation treatment side effects
- protect the body against toxic metals, such as lead and mercury
- slows the aging process

With such a good list of virtues, chlorella is high on my list of daily superfoods.

Summary

- A superfood is any natural complete food that has a high concentration of nutrients and shows health benefits beyond common food.

- Examples of superfoods: berries, turmeric, ginger, camu camu, spirulina, chlorellla.

- Turmeric root has been used for thousands of years to promote and protect health. It is safe to use of long periods of time with no toxicity.

- The key compound in turmeric is curcumin, which gives the strong, orange colour.

- Curcumin may have many properties, including anticancer, antioxidant, anti-inflammatory.

- Curcumin may work synergysically with vitamin D to increase CAMP levels that help prevent infection.

- Use turmeric powder liberally in your cooking, adding it near to the end to preserve its healing properties.

- Juice the turmeric root, along with carrot and lemon juice plus a dash of oil, for increased absorption.

- Consider supplementing with curcumin from 750–3000mg, daily depending on your health condition.

- Include more ginger in your juices, smoothie, stir-fries and even your teas.

- Camu camu is a powerful source of vitamin C. Mix some spirulina powder into your juice or smoothie for extra protein, B vitamins and iron.

- Broken cell chlorella help to mop up environmental toxins, improve your gut health, and hence your immune system.

Chapter 13
Chocolate revealed!

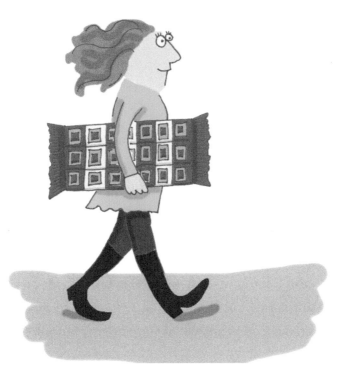

Why is chocolate good for you? Some call it a superfood. I think chocolate warrants a chapter of its own, given how important a role it plays in some women's health and happiness ... as long as it is low in sugar. The Latin name for chocolate, Theobroma cacao, means "food of the gods" for a reason. There are many documented health benefits. And I love the line, "Chocolate grows on trees, it's a plant, that makes it a vegetable, hence chocolate is good for me".

Actually, chocolate is a fruit, and whether it is good for you or not depends on how it is made. Cocoa beans contain minerals including potassium, zinc, magnesium, iron, fibre, resveratrol (antioxidant), as well as theobromine, a stimulant that acts like caffeine in some people.

It has been found that dark chocolate reduces blood pressure and helps protect the heart and arteries from damage. Researchers from Louisiana State University (2014) discovered it does this is by encouraging the growth of beneficial gut bacteria such as Bifidobacterium and lactic acid bacteria which feed on chocolate, fermenting the fibre, and producing anti-inflammatory compounds. (Ref. 1)

From pod to palate

The cocoa plant grows close to the equator, otherwise I'd have one or two in my garden! The raw cocoa pod, when split open, contains white or purple beans. The purple colour is due to resveratrol, the same health enhancing antioxidant present in grapes and wine. Also present in the untreated seed are some essential minerals as well as 54% fat, 11% protein, 31% carbohydrates, and fibre. The seeds are removed from the pod, and undergo a natural fermentation and drying process for one to two weeks. The end result is raw cocoa beans. (It's possible to now buy these raw, dried fermented cocoa beans; an acquired taste, but full of nutrients.)

A commercial chocolate manufacturer will take this dry, raw bean and dry-roast it up to 150C. This develops the colour further to brown and increases the flavour of the bean, to a taste that our modern palates expect from chocolate. The downside is that it reduces the levels of antioxidants in the cocoa. The outer shell of the bean is then removed, and the inner cocoa bean meat is broken into small pieces called "cocoa nibs." Raw cocoa nibs are made by omitting the roasting stage.

These raw cocoa nibs are delicious sprinkled on smoothies for a bit of crunch, with a nutty, slightly bitter flavour. They can also be added to a cake or muffin recipe. See the Raw Chocolate Cake Heaven recipe, where they are added to the base layer.

Cocoa nibs consist of two important components, cocoa solids and cocoa butter. In the chocolate manufacturing process, the solids are separated from the butter by pressing the nibs. The cocoa solids are then ground to a fine cocoa powder. This is the cocoa powder we use in baking. It is also used to make into commercial chocolate bars, when combined with other ingredients. Dark, bittersweet chocolates are made by adding cocoa butter, sugar, flavourings, emulsifier (usually soy lecithin, to help the ingredients blend). In the making of milk chocolate, milk is added at this stage too.

How much to eat?

Firstly, if you don't like chocolate and it does not appeal, or it makes you too jittery and stimulated, there is NO need to worry. Let's admit, it is easy to get your antioxidants elsewhere, with an abundance of rainbow-coloured vegetables and fruit. Enjoyment is the key! If, however, like me, you do love chocolate, then dark chocolate is the one to go for, with a cocoa content of 70% or more. The darker it is, the greater the content of polyphenols. They make chocolate taste bitter, so some sugar is needed to balance the bitter taste. Finding the right balance is important.

I often enjoy two to four squares of dark chocolate in the morning, aiming to savour them slowly and mindfully, and not always succeeding. It may lift your mood and combat depression, by causing an increase in serotonin and other neurotransmitters in the brain.

One of my favourite effects of chocolate consumption is a reduction in appetite. If I eat two to four small squares of dark chocolate mid-morning, I can happily make a large vegetable juice for lunch and feel satisfied. If I have too much dark chocolate i.e. four to eight squares, especially in the afternoon, I can feel discomfort from the stimulating effects of the theobromine and even experience poorer sleep that same night. It's best to determine what level of theobromine in the chocolate you can handle.

Apparently, the oldest woman on the planet, who lives in Mexico, was asked how she got to live to 127 years old. She said it was due to eating chocolate. I am pretty sure she does not mean the sugar and milk ladened variety that you and I are familiar with. David Wolfe claimed, in his Women's Wellness Conference in 2014, that chocolate (raw) is THE number one longevity food.

Some believe the health-giving benefits of chocolate are maximum when eaten as 'raw' chocolate, with higher levels of antioxidants and available nutrients. Researchers in Louisiana confirmed this when they found that the less processed the chocolate, the more able the bacteria were to produce anti-inflammatory compounds. Many raw chocolate brands are widely available online and in health food shops. I particularly like raw chocolate brands – Lovechock, Conscious Chocolate and The Raw Chocolate Company.

Try these three recipes using raw cocoa powder and raw cocoa nibs for the benefits of this superfood, with no processed sugar.

Banana Avocado Cocoa Pudding

2-3 ripe bananas
1 ripe avocado, skinned and stoned
1 tbsp cocoa powder (ideally raw)
cocoa nibs
1 medjool date (chopped) or 1tsp natural sweetener eg honey, agave syrup, maple syrup (optional)
vanilla bean or essence (optional)
optional ¼ tsp cinammon powder (optional)

- Blend all the ingredients together, adding approximately ¼ cup of water to create desired consistency, and pour into a bowl.
- Serve sprinkled with raw cocoa nibs.

Tasty cocoa trail mix

In a glass jar, mix one small handful of each of the following:

Goji berries

cocoa nibs

Omega seed mix (pumpkin, sunflower, sesame and linseed)

Keep handy and enjoy as a mid-morning snack with an apple, a cup of herb tea, or a glass of water.

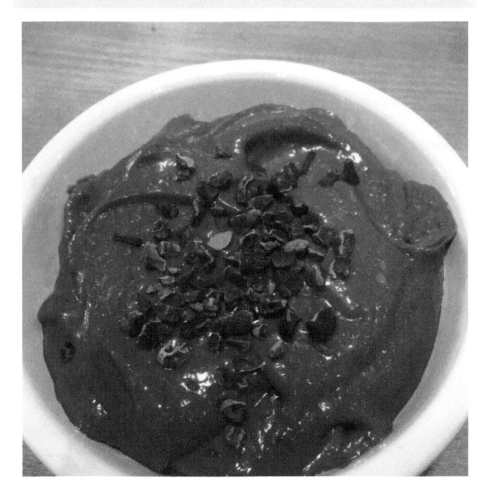

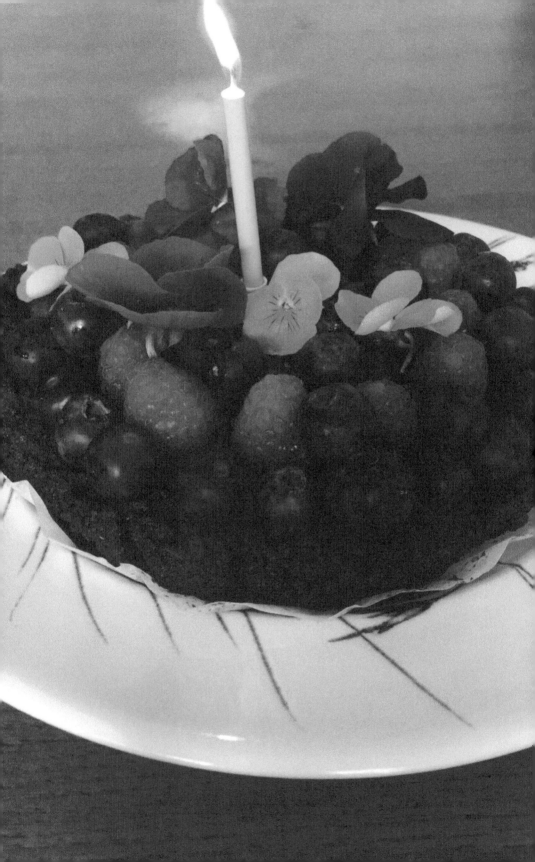

Raw Chocolate Cake Heaven
vegan, gluten-free, low sugar
(Serves approx 6-8; it is super rich, so make small slices)

Prepare a 7-8" round spring-form cake tin with a free base for ease of getting cake out in one piece. Line the tin with baking parchment. Or use a flat 9" cake plate. Quantities are approximate, unlike when making a cooked sponge cake, where quantities are crucial, so adjust to your taste.

Base
150g soaked almonds, peeled and grounded (or use ground almonds)
100g fresh medjool dates
10g cocoa powder
handful of dried sour cherries (soaked for 1 hour)
handful of cocoa nibs
1 tsp salt

Method
- Soak the almonds overnight or for a minimum of 6 hours. Drain and rinse. (Peeling the almonds is easy now, but optional).
- Grind the almonds in a food processor or nut mill.
- Blend the de-stoned dates in a processor. Add the ground almonds and salt to form a dough.
- Drain the soaked sour cherries. If needed, add some cherry soak water for a damper dough.
- Press the dough into the bottom of the tin or directly onto the flat plate to form the cake base.
- Sprinkle evenly with soaked cherries and cocoa nibs (for added crunch). Cover with cling film and leave to harden in the fridge for half an hour or longer.

Filling

2 ripe medium avocados

80g coconut oil

50g cocoa powder

50g agave nectar/maple syrup/palm sugar

1 vanilla pod beans

pinch of salt

Method

Blend all filling ingredients until smooth, like a silky chocolate mousse. Spoon this over the base and leave in fridge for one hour, or 10 minutes in freezer, if in a rush.

Topping

Top with raspberries or other fruits, chocolate curls, edible flowers, or a dusting of raw cocoa powder.

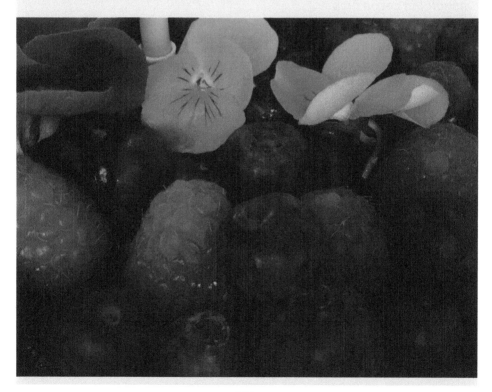

Summary

- Chocolate is actually a fruit.

- Dark chocolate may reduce blood pressure and protect the heart and arteries by encouraging beneficial gut bacteria to produce anti-inflammatory compounds.

- Chocolate contains resveratrol and other antioxidants.

- Raw cocoa nibs are produced in the manufacture of chocolate and can be eaten as a slightly bitter, yet low sugar alternative to chocolate.

- Dark chocolate is more beneficial than milk chocolate, containing less sugar and no dairy.

- Chocolate can elevate mood as it increases circulating serotonin and other neurotransmitter levels.

- Chocolate can decrease appetite.

- Adjust the amount of chocolate you consume according to how well you tolerate stimulants.

- Less processed chocolate (raw chocolate) may be more beneficial as more anti-inflammatory compounds can be produced by the gut bacteria feeding on it.

(Ref. 1)

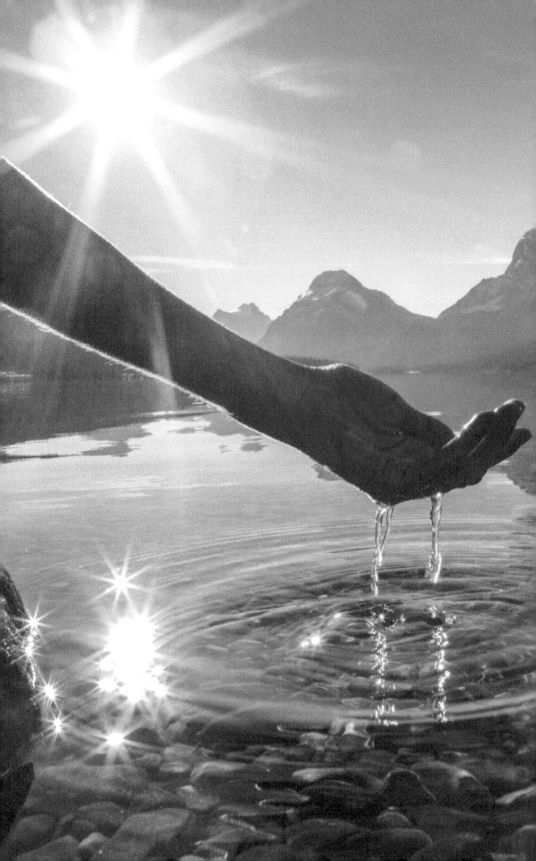

Chapter 14

Clean Living

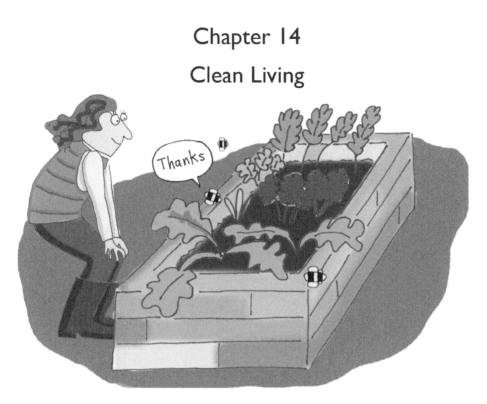

The external environment increasingly impacts our internal environment via the water we drink, the food we eat and the air we breathe, as well as what we put on our skin.

A relatively new concept, The Exposome, (Ref. 1) refers to all the complex exposures we face today, in this twenty-first century era: the tens of thousands of chemicals in our environment. Since the 1940s, at the end of World War II, we have been exposed to about 77,000 new chemicals created by the chemical industry. The industry's attitude is often "assume innocent until proven guilty". It has even been said we are the crash dummies for the chemical industry.

Eating organic food is a very important way to reduce the pollution of your body by multiple chemicals, including herbicides, pesticides and artificial fertilisers that combine and alone create serious damage right, left and centre to our cells' mitochondria. Ever wondered why you lack energy?

The manufacturers of a widely-used herbicide (containing the active ingredient glyphosate) had claimed it was completely biodegradable and safer than table salt, until earlier in 2015 when it was reclassified as a Class 2A "probable carcinogen".

Geeky science alert

Glyphosate, the active chemical widely used in some herbicides, harm the mitochondria mainly by binding with the trace mineral, manganese, making it unavailable, unable to do its normal job. Manganese is essential for the good working of an important enzyme superoxide dismutase (also known as SOD) in the mitochondria. Without SOD, many important biochemical pathways are disrupted and mitochondria dysfunction occurs, impacting our energy levels and general health.

A recent study conducted by researchers from RMIT University, published in the journal *Environmental Research* found that following an organic diet for just one week significantly reduced pesticide (commonly used in conventional food production) exposure in adults. (Ref. 2)

Xenoestrogens

These are chemicals that have an effect similar to oestrogen in our bodies and our environment. Some call this 'oestrogen pollution', creating a feminising environment, hence the name xenoestrogens.

These xenoestrogens, such as PCBs, phthalates, pesticides and DDT, all have eostrogenic effects in humans and wild animals. They are endocrine disruptors, affecting hormonal messaging in the body by imitating or enhancing the effects of eostrogens. Although banned in 1972, DDT, like its breakdown product DDE, is a xenoestrogen, which is still present in the environment.

Some present-day chemicals may be much-needed pharmaceutical drugs that save lives, others may help control the spread of disease. However, when they end up in our water supply, they can, in turn, present a massive health problem. The value of alternative methods that avoid pollution, e.g. organic farming, is a strongly debated issue.

We come into contact with xenoestrogens in four main ways:

- plastic food packaging and plastic water bottles
- pesticides on our non-organic vegetables and fruit
- nail varnish and make-up
- birth control pill

The most notorious chemical found in plastics is Bisphenol-A (BPA), which was originally created in the 1930s as a synthetic oestrogen drug. Many plastic food and drink containers that are now being produced advertise that they are BPA-free. What people in general don't know is that the BPA-free plastics that we can now buy unfortunately do not really solve the problem, as the chemicals being used to replace the discredited BPA are also oestrogenic. They are called Bisphenol B, C, D etc. and are xenoestrogens too. Research and testing is ongoing. Plastics are a big problem in our food supply; can you imagine how hard it is to buy food that has not come into contact with plastic bags, plastic containers, cling film wrap, or even the plastic lining of tins e.g. tinned tomatoes?

Non-organic meat and dairy products contain chlorine and hormone residues, which can have estrogenic effects. In men, the eostrogenic environment may result in declining sperm quality or fertility rates. In women, it may lead to an epidemic of female diseases, including some types of breast cancer, fibrocystic breast disease, uterine fibroids, ovarian cysts, all traceable to excess eostrogen/deficient progesterone.

The liver has a massive job detoxifying the body, acting as a filter and protecting us from the harmful effects of environmental toxins as well as internally made substances e.g. endogenous oestrogen that also needs to be removed from the body. Anything that impairs liver function or ties up the detoxifying function will result in excess eostrogen levels. Remember to take care of your liver.

Time to Detox

Some detoxification solutions have been discussed earlier in this book. Here's a checklist:

- Eat a rainbow of organic fruit and vegetables; make meat your side dish.

- Increase your fibre intake (Chapter 2, pg 32) to enable oestrogen molecules to be carried out of the body via the colon.

- Perform moderate aerobic exercise (see Section 2, 'DANCE'). Research shows that physical activity curtails overproduction of oestrogen. It also enables some toxins to be excreted via sweat.

- Drink enough filtered water to create clear pee.

- Twice a year, do a juice 'fast' for one day or even up to a week, ideally around the spring and autumn equinox.

- Take chlorella tablets. This tiny single-celled algae binds with heavy metals and some pesticides, and helps remove them from the body.

Here are the chemical names of a few main xenoestrogens to watch out for:

- Parabens (methylparaben, ethylparaben, propylparaben and butylparaben) commonly used as a preservative

- Bisphenol A (BPA) banned in EU and US for use in baby bottles

- Bisphenol S (BPS)

- Phthalates in plastics

- BHA food preservative

How to avoid xenoeostrogens

- Choose organic, locally grown, in-season food; loose and fresh, not wrapped in plastic

- Minimise use of non-organic fruit and vegetables

- Buy food in glass jars to avoid some exposure to the plastic-lined tins e.g. tomato passata. The acidic nature of the tomato juice possibly reacts with the plastic lining, causing further leaching of BPA into tinned tomatoes.

- Reduce use of plastics as much as possible; instead, use glass and ceramics

- Don't refill plastic water bottles. Buy a good quality drinking bottle.   My favourite is a glass water bottle called i9 Informed Water Bottle (see 'Resources').

- Use chlorine-free and unbleached paper products e.g. coffee filters, tampons etc.

- Filter your drinking water with a high-quality filter, reverse osmosis system, or by distillation.

- Avoid all cosmetics that have added parabens.

- Use shampoos and toothpastes free from sodium lauryl sulfate and parabens.

- Avoid most perfumes, unless made from essential oils. I love to use lavender, patchouli or rose essential oil.

To avoid chemicals in the home, choose your laundry and household cleaning products with care. Some products that I like to use are made by Ecover, Bio-D and Libby Chan (see 'Resources').

Alternatively, make your own! There are many easy to follow instructions in Janey Lee Grace's book, *Imperfectly Natural Woman*, using simple ingredients like lemon, white vinegar and bicarbonate of soda!

Chapter 15
Making changes - one mouthful at a time

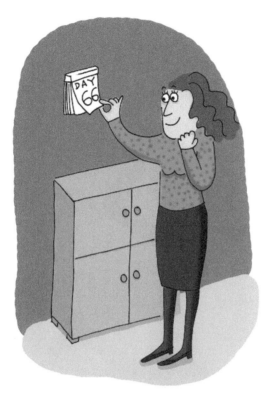

If you are feeling overwhelmed with all the sometimes conflicting information out there ... BUT know you want to make changes to feel well and improve your energy, prevent chronic disease from starting, or slow down chronic disease progression, here's a few simple steps to follow.

Ease into this gently, developing new habits, adding new foods and supplements as you go. Make simple changes to start with. Become interested in a long-term shift in consciousness.

"The journey
of a
thousand miles
begins with
one step."

Lao Tzu   6th–5th century BC

In supporting a client in reversing heart disease, it became clear to her that she could make the changes to her diet as long as:

1. She did not feel hungry
2. She liked the food

This gave her a good framework for success. I think this applies to most of us. Now you ask yourself, "What would be your requirements to make a dietary change successful and sustainable?"

There is a common belief, originating in the work of Maxwell Maltz when he published *Psycho-Cybernetics* in 1960, which says that it takes 21 days to form a new habit. This, apparently, is not true. Phillippa Lally, psychology researcher at University of London, exposed this myth in a study following 96 people over a 12-week period. She found that, on average, it takes 66 days to change a habit, and can vary greatly from person to person.

Rather than being disheartened by this, I feel it's good to realise that permanent change can be a long, slow road. It's best to embrace a longer timeline that is permanent. Allow for relapses; include them. They do not mean that you are failing, it is human nature. Celebrate not being perfect.

When it comes to making changes to how and what you eat, many experts on this subject recognise that it is not a question of willpower. In *The Yoga of Eating*, Charles Eisenstein says, "Reliance on willpower reveals a profound distrust of oneself." And, "Life becomes a constant regime of 'shoulds' and 'shouldn'ts'." I remember, at different times in my life, attempting to lose weight and saying the famous line when I failed at my daily plan: "I'll start again tomorrow."

Later in life, I was aware of the polarity of opposing desires when I was attempting to eat a largely raw vegan diet. Some days, it worked and I felt good physically and emotionally. Other days, I found myself feeling tired and craving and succumbing to the delights of cooked food.

It was not until about five years later when I had changed my career from school teacher to Nia dancer and teacher, and felt a new facet of myself emerging, with greater self-expression and vitality, that I could effortlessly make changes to my eating style and habit, and celebrate the continuous evolution, not just of my dietary choices, but of the whole of me. Without consciously knowing it, my ultimate aim has been to integrate my body and my soul so that what I actually want to eat is what my body needs.

Eisenstein expresses this beautifully: "A discrepancy between what we eat and who we are in the world generates a kind of tension, which is resolved either when the diet moves back in line with the person's incarnate role, or when the person's entire life changes to come into harmony with the new diet." Nothing about you is separate; your body and emotions and mind are all related, so when you change one thing, you are affecting everything. My experience echoes this, and now I find it effortless to avoid certain foods that I know make me feel unwell, such as sugar, in a way that was impossible for me 15 years ago.

Here are the steps to follow if you find yourself feeling overwhelmed.

This *five stages of change process* may empower you with your changes. As you read through my example of these five stages, imagine your own scenario. (Ref. 1) Then try it out substituting in your own example. It goes like this for me:

Stage I: Identify a Problem – "What problem?"

Err, am I feeling tired and lethargic? I want more energy? Mmm, is it even possible to do all I want to do in a day, or are my expectations too high? What could I accomplish in a day with more energy? I wonder...

Stage 2: Mull it over – "What's possible, pros and cons?"

Could changing my diet make any difference to my energy levels? How about actually looking at what I eat to find out if there is something that is draining my energy? I could give up eating wheat, see how I feel. But what would I have for lunch? A normal bread sandwich is so easy and convenient.

Stage 3: Get ready – "How can I change?" Plans, structures and support

Ok, I am going to begin on Monday, tomorrow, and cut out all wheat and wheat-containing products for three weeks. Now I am going to decide, with the help of recipe books, what I am going to make for lunch. I will prepare a menu for the next seven days and repeat it for three weeks. I could make soup the day before so that it is easy to warm up at lunchtime. I could buy some gluten-free bread or crackers that I like. I am going to ask my friend to do it with me, so we can support each other.

Stage 4: Off we go – "I am doing it!"

Already been on this zero-wheat plan for two weeks now. Lunch is great; I just had a large, green vegetable juice with half an avocado blended into it. Then I ate carrot and celery sticks dipped in hummus. Feeling really full and satisfied. Tomorrow for lunch, I am having a vegetable soup that I have already made. This is exciting. And I don't feel that "after lunch" sleepiness.

Stage 5: Keep going – "It's just the way I am now"

I can't imagine how I survived eating all that bread, not to mention cakes and biscuits. I never even realised how sleepy it made me feel. I am not even tempted. And it gets easier and easier. I just need to look at these wheat products to be reminded, and know how it would make me feel. Oh, and there are other treats that do the trick, like a walk with my dog across the fields, the wind blowing us along, celebrating the elements. Or taking a 20-minute break to read my novel.

"Falling off the Wagon" can happen at any time; it's not the end of the world, just a reminder of how eating wheat seriously does not work for me, and I cannot wait to get back to the new way, starting right now!

How does it go for you?

Exercise to develop a new habit:

Choose an example in your life situation where you have already succeeded in making changes, and run through the five stages, imagining the whole process. Write it all down. Become familiar with the stages.

Then choose an aspect you want to change and record the stages as you go through them.

Now, begin it!

Summary

- Make simple changes first that you can live with. Take one step at a time.

- Leave behind the 'shoulds' and 'shouldn'ts'.

- Instead of relying on willpower, make lifestyle changes so that the whole of you is changing, not just your diet. Then there is more harmony and less need for willpower.

- Use the five stages if it appeals to you.

- A relapse can happen and does not mean failure, rather a reminder of what did not work.

(Ref. 1)

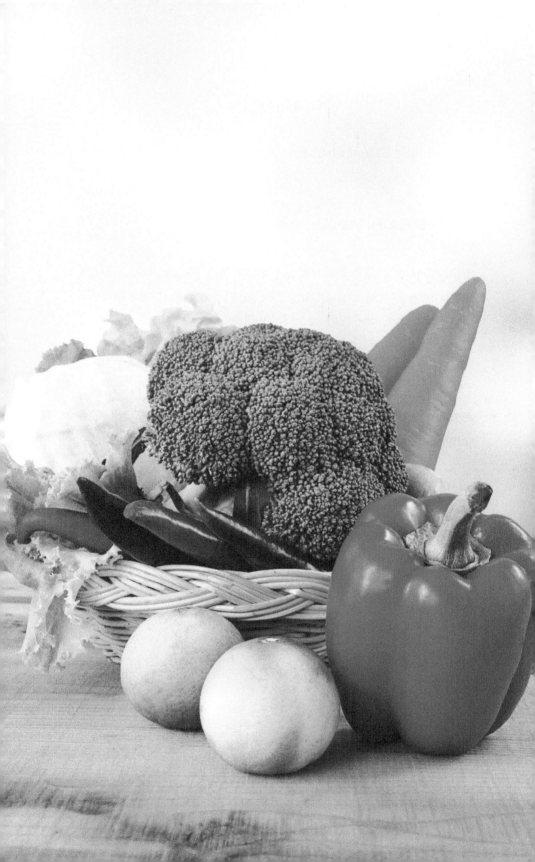

Chapter 16
Meal ideas

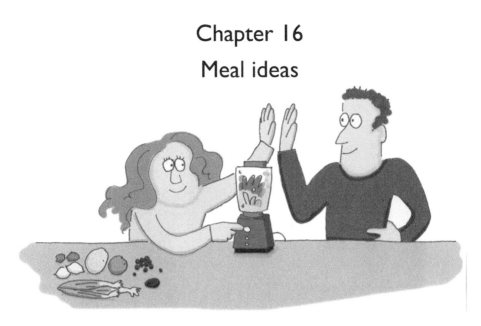

Here are a few meal ideas to stimulate your creativity. It's time to take action, that is easy and positive. There is something even joyous about accomplishing lifestyle and dietary changes that makes you feel more energised and vibrant.

Breakfast ideas

Delay breakfast so that you have not eaten anything for 16 to 18 hours between your evening meal and your first food of the day ... break-fast. This is commonly know as Intermittent Fasting, and is a variation on the 5:2 diet. I find this variation more appealing. It means the pounds can drop off effortlessly, or stay off (if you have no weight to lose), while you sleep. So if you ended your last meal at 7 p.m., then have your first food of the day between 11 a.m. and 1 p.m. Water, herb teas and even green tea are fine before eating. I even drink coconut water mixed with a green 'superfood' powder at around 8 a.m., before I leave to teach my Nia class at 8.45 a.m. If you exercise during this time, before breakfast, for at least 30 minutes, the weight loss and health benefits are increased.

Remember, it's not necessary to eat breakfast as soon as you get out of bed. You choose when to 'break' your 'fast'.

Make a Green Smoothie

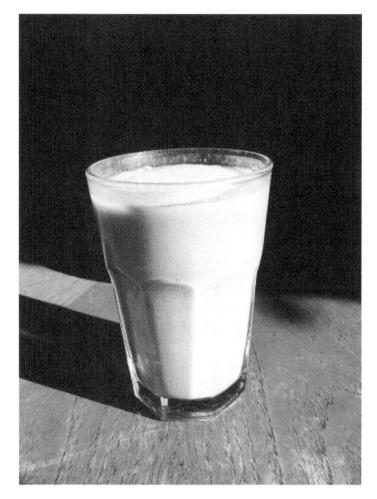

Green smoothies are a wonderfully nutritious way to start the day. (Also great for a fast snack or meal replacement.) They are adaptable and variable. Generally, they include some ripe fruit, some soft, green leaves, and some water, coconut water or nut milk. You can add a variety of spices and superfoods that you enjoy, to add flavour and nutrients. Some fruits work better than others.

The combinations are endless. Have fun experimenting!

Here are my preferred ingredients. Use one type from each of the three groups, or a combination, and blend with enough water to make the smoothie to your required consistency:

1. Ripe fruit

banana

pear

berries

pineapple

mango

2. Greens

baby spinach

watercress

rocket

baby lettuce leaves

romaine leaves

celery

3. Spices and superfoods

cinnamon

vanilla

green powder

spirulina powder

ground linseed

barley grass powder

broccoli sprout powder

cocoa powder

dessicated coconut

Or if you prefer to follow a Green Smoothie recipe:

Green Banana Smoothie

Blend

- 2 ripe banana
- 1 tbsp freshly ground linseeds
- a handful of baby spinach or 1 stick of celery
- 1 tsp spirulina powder
- water or coconut water, to desired consistency

Option:

Sprinkle with raw cocoa nibs.

Many more smoothie recipes can be found on the Internet and in recipe books.

And here are two breakfast ideas already mentioned earlier

Mega green vegetable juice (Chapter 5)
'Berry tasty breakfast' recipe (Chapter 3)

Snack ideas for mid-morning and mid-afternoon

- carrot sticks
- hummus
- a handful of soaked nuts
- apple dipped in nut butter
- a fresh vegetable juice
- a smoothie

Lunch ideas

- A large and colourful salad, including a selection of green leaves (lettuce, rocket, watercress, baby spinach), cherry tomatoes, avocado, carrot sticks, or grated cucumber.

- A large green smoothie

- Mega green vegetable juice blended with ½ an avocado or ½ cup of almond milk

- Home-made vegetable soup

- Non-vegetarian option – tinned sardines (sustainable source), cheese (organic and unpasteurised, if possible) with salad.

Dinner ideas

Salads - vegetarian ideas

- Middle Eastern salad is one of my favourites – see recipe in Chapter 8.

- Steamed vegetables dressed with olive oil, lemon juice, sea salt and pepper

- Cooked grain – choose a gluten-free grain (maybe try one you are not familiar with, from the following: brown basmati rice, quinoa, millet, buckwheat or amaranth).

- Bean dishes can be hearty and filling, great comfort food – recipe below.

- Oven 'roasted' vegetables – recipe to follow.

Recipe

Sweet potato, lentil and white haricot bean stew

Serves 3-4

- 1 onion, sliced
- 1-2 large sweet potato, sliced
- ½ cup red lentils
- 1 cup haricot beans, dry or tinned
- 2 cloves garlic, sliced
- 200g long green beans, cut into thirds
- ½ red chilli, sliced thinly
- 1 tsp Marigold bouillon
- small handful of parsely, chopped
- drizzle of olive oil
- sea salt and pepper, to taste

Method

If using dry haricot beans, place in boiling water and simmer for approximately two hours until soft and cooked.

Meanwhile in another pan, add the sliced onion, garlic and sweet potato to 1-2 cm hot water and simmer a few minutes. Add the lentils along with 500 ml water and the bouillon. Allow to simmer, adding more water if needed, as the lentils absorb the water when cooking. After about 20 minutes, add the green beans, chilli and cooked haricot beans. Cook for a further 6-7 minutes. Add the parsely, season, and serve drizzled with olive oil. Great with a green salad!

Beans and wind

If you have trouble with flatulence when eating beans, it is likely to be caused by two things:

- the increase in fibre which your digestion is not used to
- the complex sugars called alpha-galactosides in the beans which the human body has no enzymes to digest

Soaking has no effect on flatulence, according to bean expert Gregory Gray. Apparently, if you eat beans more frequently, your microflora adjusts and less gas is produced. Gregory, who has been studying beans for 10 years at the U. S. Department of Agriculture's Western Regional Research lab in Albany, Calififornia, says, "In cultures that routinely eat beans, you don't hear a lot of complaining about flatulence."

Whether you use dried beans or ready-cooked beans, from a tin or carton, depends mainly on how much time you have to cook.

Some say dried beans must be soaked, others say soaking dried beans reduces their flavour and texture.

Here's two methods:

1. Soak dried beans in three times their volume of water, for 6 hours or overnight. Then cooked for approximately 1.5 to 2 hours.

2. Or miss the soaking stage and cook dried unsoaked beans, by adding boiling water to them in a pan, not cold water at the start. Then simmer them, covered with a lid, for about 2 hours.

Recipe:
Oven 'roasted' vegetables

Serves 4

- 500g potatoes
- 2-3 sweet potatoes, cut into wedges of similar size
- 4 carrots, sliced 1cm thick
- 2 onions, sliced
- 1 of each: red pepper, yellow pepper and green pepper, seeded and quartered
- 5 cloves of garlic, sliced thinly
- thyme and oregano, pinch of dry or sprig of fresh
- water, enough to cover tray 1cm deep
- 2 tbsp balsamic vinegar (optional)
- a good drizzle of olive oil
- sea salt and black pepper

Mix the vegetables well, in a shallow roasting tray. Cook in the oven at 180°C for 20-30 minutes until the potatoes are ready. Keep checking and adding small amounts of water, if the tray dries out, to allow the vegetables to steam, and protect the olive oil.

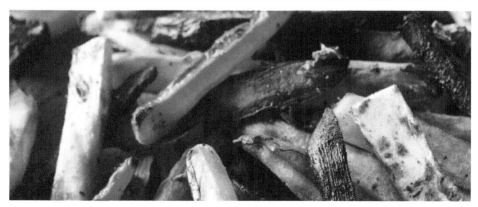

Pudding ideas

Depending how well you deal with 'sugar' will determine how often you make a pudding and how much sweetener (honey, agave syrup, coconut palm sugar, date syrup, maple syrup) you add.

Some people need to watch their sugar intake and keep it low if they have developed insulin resistance (reduced sensitivity to insulin). Let's not forget ... plain and simple fruit makes a wonderful dessert, slices of pineapple, a bunch of grapes or sliced oranges sprinkled with chopped almonds etc.

Then there are the times when only a pudding will do. Here are two of my favourites; they are delicious, quick to make, involve no cooking, and provide abundant nutrients.

Apple with Raspberry Super Sauce

- Finely chop an apple.
- Blend a cup of frozen raspberries with 2 tbsp freshly ground linseeds and enough water or coconut water to make a sauce.
- Pour sauce over apples and top with chopped pre-soaked almonds.

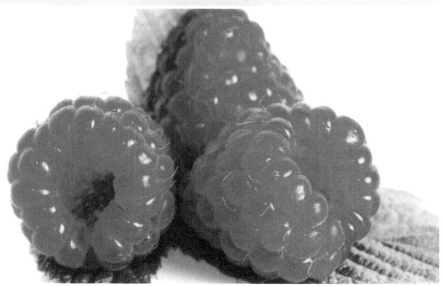

Choc Berry Balls

This sweet treat comes close to being a truffle.

- 1 cup raisins
- ½ cup cranberries
- ¼ cup sour cherries
- ½ cup dried apricots
- 1 cup almonds, freshly ground (ideally soaked, rinsed and dried, before grinding)
- ½ cup chia seeds
- 3 tbsp raw cocoa powder
- approx ½ cup Agave syrup

Method

- Blend raisins until soft and add the ground almonds in the food processor.
- Mix well.
- Add cranberries and sour cherries and blend further.
- Finally add cocoa powder, chia seeds and agave syrup, and blend until a soft ball forms.
- Mould into about 30 small balls, roll in cocoa butter, or leave as they are.

Chapter 17
Taking stock

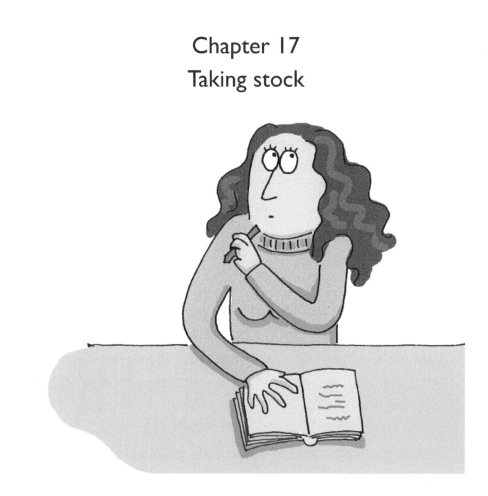

Finally ... take three deep breaths and acknowledge how far you have come. To support you in taking stock of what you have read and absorbed so far, here's a few question related to each chapter.

Exercise

Rather than write in this book, you can download a worksheet for this exercise from the website.

Here we go!

1. **Have you tried the body sway** or the awareness exercise to
   awaken your inner guru?
Are you more in touch with what your body needs and does not
   need?
What have you learned about yourself?
Make some notes here:

2. **Are you eating more plants?**
Have you increased your fibre intake?
Have you tried grinding linseeds and taking them every day?
What changes have you observed in your body, your digestion,
   your elimination?

3. **Have you been aware of eating more colours in your fruits
   and vegetables?**
Have you made more colourful salads and eaten more berries?

4. **Assess how many glasses of wine you drink a week.**
Remember there are other ways to get the antioxidant,
   resveratrol. What are they?
What changes are you committed to making here?

5. Do you have a way of making juice?

Is the equipment out and ready to go?

Or is it hidden at the back of a cupboard?

How often, per week, can you promise yourself to make a healthy
vegetable juice?

6. Have you tried soaking some nuts or seeds?

Sprinkling them onto a salad?

Have you made some nut milk?

Are you substituting this nut milk to decrease your dairy intake?

**7. Are you getting your omega-3s from vegetarian or fish
sources?**

Have you included coconut oil in your diet?

Are you reducing your intake of vegetable oils to get a healthier
ratio of omega-6 to omega-3?

8. What new 'uncooked' recipe have you tried?

Which new grains have you tried?

Have you reduced the amount of times you start a recipe with
frying an onion?

Have you tried 'simmer-frying' instead?

9. What fermented food are you eating this week?

Have you made any sauerkraut yet? This recipe works!

10. What supplements do you take? List them here.

Do any of them contain undesirable additives?

Check the labels.

Can you find alternatives?

Or do you choose, instead, to make and drink a vegetable juice
each day?

11. Do you know what your Vitamin D level is?

Are you taking a Vitamin D supplement?

Are you eating more greens? Are you taking a Vitamin K2
supplement?

**12. List here the superfoods you are taking and congratulate
yourself!**

**13. How dark is your taste in chocolate? Cultivate a taste for less
sweet, darker chocolate. You only need a little. Less is more!**

With one small square of dark chocolate, sit down and take five
minutes to eat it mindfully. What did you notice?

14. List here how you have reduced your use of plastic food:

How else are you avoiding xenoestrogens in your home?

15. Acknowledge the changes you have made and congratulate yourself, again.

What are your change challenges?

16. List one new thing you are going to make this week for each mealtime:

- breakfast
- mid-morning snack
- lunch
- mid-afternoon snack
- dinner

NOW

Choose any idea that appeals to you, when you are ready, whatever looks easiest, most appealing, and make a start.

As I love to say in Nia classes, "Do it your body's way; only you know what feels best for your body."

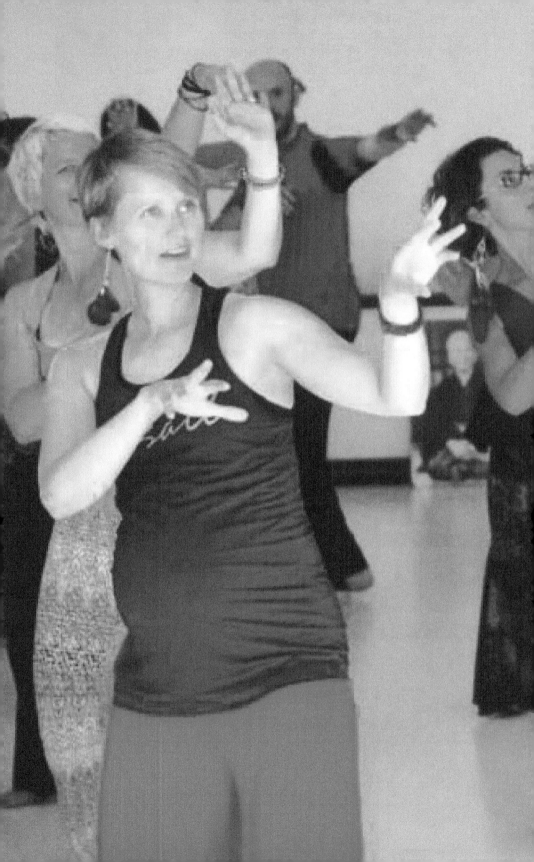

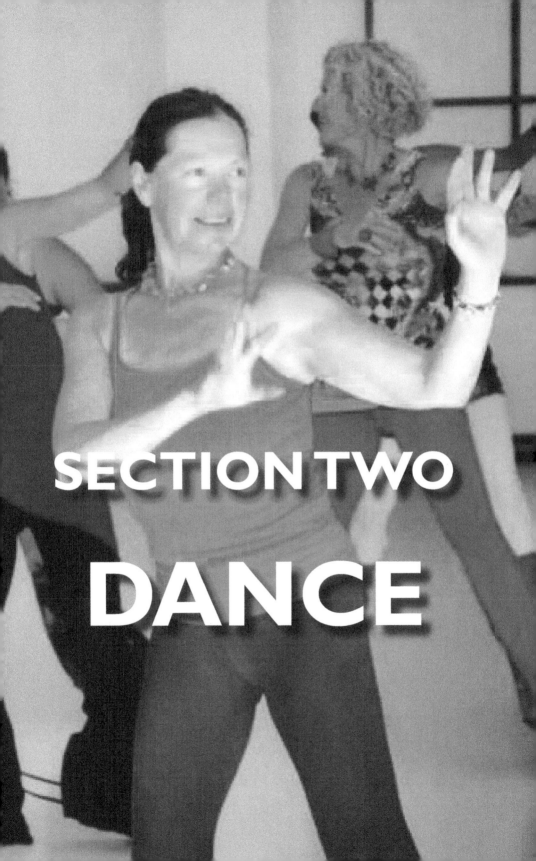

SECTION TWO

DANCE

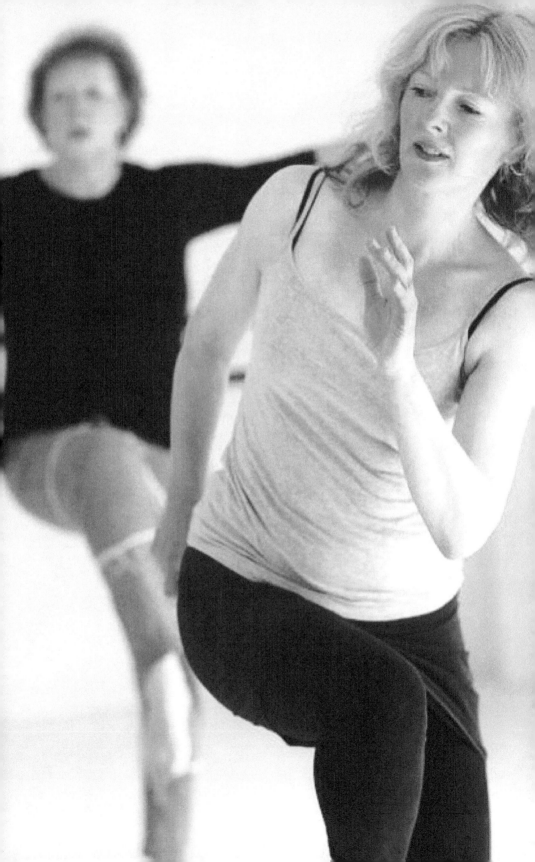

SECTION 2: DANCE

Let's first take a general look at the value of exercise.

Chapter 1
Exercise – Why bother?

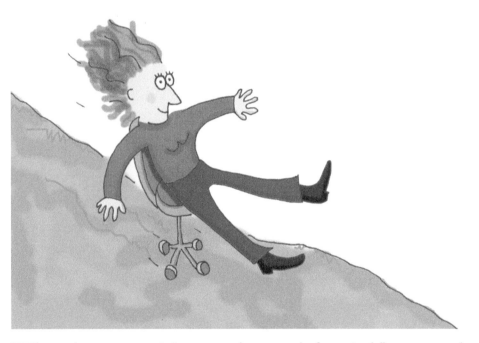

These days, we are sitting more than ever before. And "you cannot be truly well at the same time as being unfit," says Dr Doug Graham, raw athletic coach.

We sit on chairs to work at computers, to travel, to be entertained, and to eat. We were designed to move. There is no wonder that we are now a modern species who have chronic and acute back problems, joint problems, obesity problems and heart problems, as well as depression.

Lack of movement plays a big part in all of this, although, of course, nutrition and emotional health are interrelated too.

Have you heard of brown fat? We all have it in varying amounts, usually between our shoulder blades and along our spine. Unlike regular ol' white fat, which stores calories, mitochondria-packed brown-fat cells are calorie-burning and heat producing.

All babies are born with it, enabling the baby to keep warm. Brown fat reduces with age and is likely to be a main reason why we put on weight as we age. Exercise increases the amount and activity of brown fat and can even turn 'bad' white fat into brown fat. (Ref. 1) Another reason to exercise!

Energy Boosting Tip
from Ann Davies, retired doctor

"I swear by Epsom salts in a bath for an energy boost. Dissolve at least 350g in a hot bath, and stay in the bath for about 30 minutes. Epsom salts contain magnesium sulphate, which studies have shown to be effectively absorbed through the skin under these conditions. I experience an increase in energy about 3 hours later, which lasts for roughly 12 hours. Magnesium is also good for muscle relaxation. A 25kg bag of Epsom salts is a good investment. I feel that it's important to buy the pharmaceutical grade, in order to minimise impurities."

The following three studies show us what we know makes common sense; "move it or lose it".

1 Researchers at Cambridge University were involved in a study following an impressively large group; 300,000 European men and women over a 12-year period. Their physical activity as well as their weight and obesity levels were recorded. Prof. Ekelund concluded from this study in early 2015, that "the greatest risk [of early death] was in those classed inactive". Researchers went on to say eliminating inactivity in Europe would cut mortality rates by nearly 7.5% but interestingly eliminating obesity would cut rates by only 3.6%. He says, "20 minutes of physical activity every day is all that is needed to transform your health, a brisk walk!" (Ref. 2)

2 In a cancer prevention paper, Graham A. Colditz said, "Breast cancer risk factors such as obesity and physical inactivity will never be eliminated completely; but ... we could still prevent thousands of cases of breast cancer each year." And, "Women who are active during both youth and adulthood may have a lower risk of premenopausal and postmenopausal breast cancer than women who are inactive or active during only one of these phases of life." (Ref. 3)

3 In an inspiring article called *Seeing exercise as the best medicine*, Dr John Mandrola describes a study (Ref. 4 and 5) in which 12 sedentary human volunteers take part in a one-year training program. These volunteers started by exercising for 30 to 45 minutes three to four times per week by brisk walking, jogging, swimming, or cycling. By the end of the study, the average exercise time was seven to nine hours per week. The results were striking. They found that healthy people who made a commitment to exercise regularly developed cardiac changes normally only seen in elite-level athletes.

Mandrola also describes one of his own patients with high blood pressure and arrhythmia of the heart, who took his advice to start exercising. He began slowly, just with walking. Amazingly, results showed changes not just to the heart! "Glucose metabolism improved, brain function sharpened, and mitochondria grew more efficient. Seemingly overnight, an unhealthy person became healthy."

He ends the article with the reminder:

"We only have one heart
and one body
and one life.
Health needs to be
a priority choice."

Movement is vital to our health. Some of us are not particularly drawn to it, and quite frankly would like to spend the rest of our lives on the sofa, preferably eating! Other individuals can't sit still, and spend much of their life buzzing about being highly active, but also verge on being overstressed. Once again, finding balance is vital. You will know roughly where you fit along that spectrum of activity type.

Chapter 2
Changing exercise habits

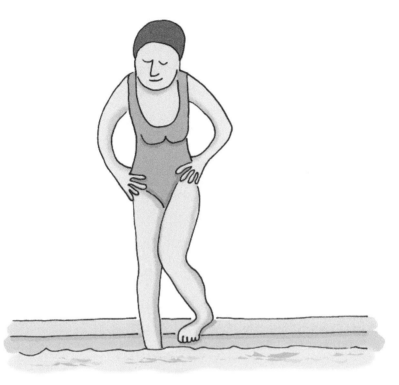

I have come to realise that rather than rely on willpower, with its limited 'battery life', I would rather find an activity that I really enjoy and want to take part in, several times a week. As a young person, I always loved to dance, and I spent many years being an enthusiastic horsewoman, competing and captaining my university team. However, there has also been quite a phlegmatic side to my nature too. This gave me the tendency to be sedentary, spending many hours reading or knitting.

As I grew older, the requirement for more movement grew and I started to cultivate and develop a more active quality. For a few years, I enjoyed rebounding on a mini trampoline.

This is not only a good workout for the muscles, but also wonderful for lymphatic drainage, aiding the body in detoxifying.

Energy Boosting Tip
from Tamara Donn, EFT Trainer, Master Trainer
www.transformationforwomen.co.uk

"First thing in the morning, I like to spend 20 minutes dancing on my rebounder (small trampoline) to a playlist of my all-time favourite upbeat tracks. Although most mornings I look forward to this, there are times when I feel tired or simply not in the mood. Then I am gentle with myself and either dance for less time or simply jog slowly on the rebounder. I always feel better, have more energy and feel ready for my day."

Then I discovered Nia, a holistic fitness practice, and this fulfilled most of my exercise needs (see Chapter 3, 'Nia'). I also love to walk. I encourage you to find one or two activities or types of exercise that you enjoy and that suits your personality and ability.

A good place to start is to acknowledge where you are. Without judgement, review all that you have done and not done in the area of exercise over the last months and years, and take a fresh look at how to add more exercise. Then formulate an action plan that is enjoyable and sustainable. Remember that what you do most days is important, not what you do once in a while.

Start by ask yourself two simple questions:

1. What exercise do I enjoy?

2. What is practically possible with my current lifestyle and physical condition?

Here's an example of my train of thought as I took a look at my situation:

- I like to swim, but I really don't like being immersed in heavily chlorinated water, inhaling chlorine fumes and smelling it on my skin and hair for hours afterwards. I also dislike getting wet and then going outside in the winter. I sometimes find it quite boring. That rules out swimming.

- I am not very competitive and really don't like going to the gym. So no competitive sports, no gym.

- Mornings are the best times for me to be active.

- Walking is wonderful, but unless I have a dog that needs walking, I don't make it a priority and so don't get around to it.

Now go through your own investigation to see what works and does not work for you.

We are all unique. What are you drawn to? Whether it be a competitive sport, swimming, walking, dancing, the gym, yoga or martial arts, the main point is to begin and make it a regular practice, just like brushing your teeth.

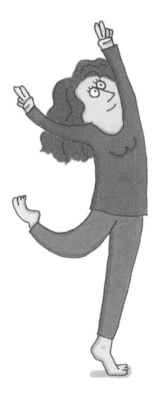
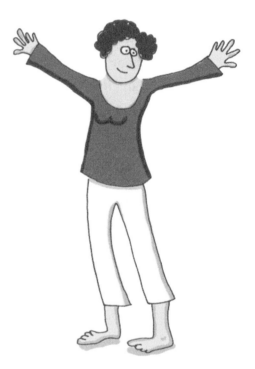

Chapter 3
Nia

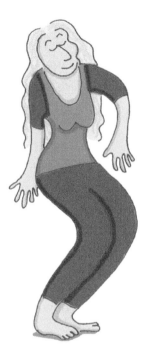

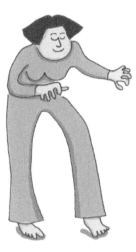

Firstly, let's look at dance

I love to dance. I have been dancing since the age of five when I gave a spontaneous free-flowing dance performance to Mozart in front of elderly relatives in New York. Dancing is one of my passions. Like many young girls, I took ballet, tap and modern dance lessons, but never felt particularly gifted or successful there.

This experience did not stop me from enjoying disco dancing as a teenager. Quite frankly, I have never since stopped dancing.

There are many physical and mental health benefits for people of all ages:

- improves strength, flexibility and endurance
- keeps muscles and joints active
- conditions heart and lungs
- strengthens bones and reduces risk of osteoporosis
- improves balance and spatial awareness
- increases self-esteem and confidence
- enhances self-expression and social skills

Recently, over 400 studies in the field of neuroscience have revealed that dance actually bulks up the brain by growing new brain cells. This means that your ability to acquire knowledge and actually think increases. Consequently, the brain that 'dances' is changed by it.

And dancing also increases the brain's neuroplasticity, the ability of neurons to re-wire and grow new connections. (Ref. 6) If you already love to dance, I don't think you need any more convincing, and if you are not sure about dancing, think again ...

People the world over enjoy expressing themselves through movement. There are so many different forms of movement and dance to choose from: ballroom, tango, salsa, Nia, Zumba, 5Rhythms, to name but a few. It's about giving them a go and tasting each one, rather like ice cream flavours; see which appeals, until you find your favourite.

What is Nia?

Simply put, Nia cardio-dance fitness classes combine moves from the dance arts, the martial arts and the healing arts – for the benefit of body, mind, emotions and spirit.

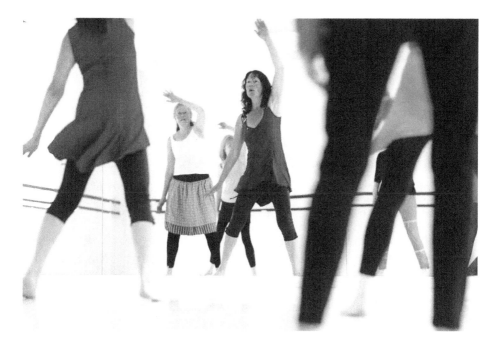

It is my most favourite form of movement and dance. I have been practicing Nia several times a week for the last ten years, and teaching Nia for the last nine years. It has changed my life, my body and my relationship with my body!

It's a grounded, low-impact cardiovascular fitness class that teaches you to move Joyfully, be expressive and feel more Alive in your body. A word about 'Joy'; it is used here and in Nia's first principle *The Joy of Movement* to describe a life-force vibration, a somatic experience of aliveness, that is different from feeling joy or being happy. So there is no pressure to feel joyous while doing Nia, it can be done in any mood.

It's drawn from three styles of dance (jazz, modern and Duncan dance), three martial arts (tai chi, tae kwon so, aikido) and three healing arts (yoga, the Feldenkrais Method, the Alexander Technique). Nia involves a variety of movement speeds, styles, ranges of motion and energy dynamics. (Ref. 7) Regardless of age, gender, or physical ability, Nia is adaptable for everybody, whether you feel out of shape, uncoordinated or indeed supremely athletic. In my classes, students' ages range widely from mid-twenties to eighty-three. A truly mixed ability class!

Nia is done barefoot

Why barefoot? In order to strengthen and increase flexibility of the foot and ankle joint, to sense the soles, the heel and the ball of the foot, as well as to improve balance and stability. Nia creates happy malleable feet. I am grateful for my increasingly strong feet as I dance through life enjoying every twist and turn!

Yet it's more than dance, more than an exercise class. "Nia becomes a moving meditation due to its focus on staying in the moment," says physician and black belt Nia teacher, Carrie Magill.

Nia has been practiced internationally since the early 1980s. The founder and co-creator, Debbie Rosas, says that Nia moves are based on what she calls, "The Body's Way". That is, the design and function of the body. "I believe that self-healing is a birthright and that given the right kind of movement as medicine, anybody can feel better". And after all, isn't that what we are all aiming for?

Debbie also says, "Nia's philosophy and approach to movement has grown out of thousands of people's experiences following The Body's Way map to understand how to use their body more functionally in order to feel better, self-heal and condition the body." Nia is now described as "a design system for sustainability of the body."

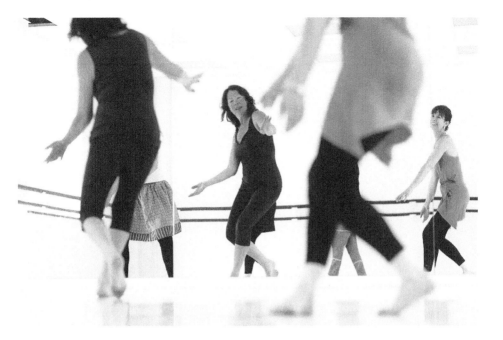

The class is a blend of form and freedom, a blend of choreography and 'freedance', of yin and yang. Even within the choreography, everyone's dance is unique. And since 2007 when I found my first Nia class, with Nia trainer Dorit Noble, my body and indeed my relationship with my body, has changed beyond recognition. I have grown fitter, slimmer and dropped at least two dress sizes. More than anything, my awareness has increased. I notice how I walk, sit, get up from a chair, and I am grateful for still being able to sit on the floor with ease. This enables me to understand why elderly yogis in India can sit on mats for hours when old men and women of our Western culture have a real problem even picking something up off the floor.

I often hear students say they come to Nia not only to keep fit, but also because it makes them feel less stressed and more happy with a sense of being alive, energised, yet centred and mindful.

Nia Moving to Heal classes are also available, which turn movement into a therapeutic experience, to support people, specifically who are in recovery, in dealing with injury, trauma, grief and short- or long-term illness.

Just as 'reading the menu' is not the same as 'eating the food', I recommend you find a class near you and sense, even taste, the experience; give it a go! To find a class near you, visit www.nianow.com where there are classes listed in 45 different countries. You can also join the online Nia community on Facebook at TheNiaTechniqueUK. If you live too far from a class, there are Nia DVDs available online to use at home.

What Nia students say about Michele's classes

Lynette Malitski

"I'm an eighty-year-old, awaiting heart surgery, and I wake up on a Tuesday with a singing heart, knowing that my Nia class will bring energy, happiness and a positive feeling to my day. Although I'm short of puff, I'm able to join in at my own level and lose myself in the music."

Sophie Aldred

"Nia is quite simply the highlight of my week. Whatever way I'm being when I walk in, I skip out taller, stronger, more connected with myself and the group, and ready for anything!"

Judith Silver

"I'm so grateful to have discovered Nia, and to have the good fortune to live near Michele so I can attend her classes. I love the invitation to listen to my body and adapt the practice to suit my needs exactly, knowing it will be different every time and that's how it should be. I love Michele's gentle and joyous way of sharing the movements and ideas. I was also lucky enough to get to do the White Belt training a couple of years ago, and that brings an extra layer of enjoyment and identification to the classes for me."

Judi Holmes

"Where else can I dance and prance to my heart's content and feel the love and freedom that I can express, along with other women. It's a great feeling."

Lin Serlin

"Nia is fun, offers freedom of movement and fantastic joy! An uplifting way to exercise and move my body! Free the inner dancer with Nia. And Michele is amazing – she brings light, joy and passion to the whole Nia experience!"

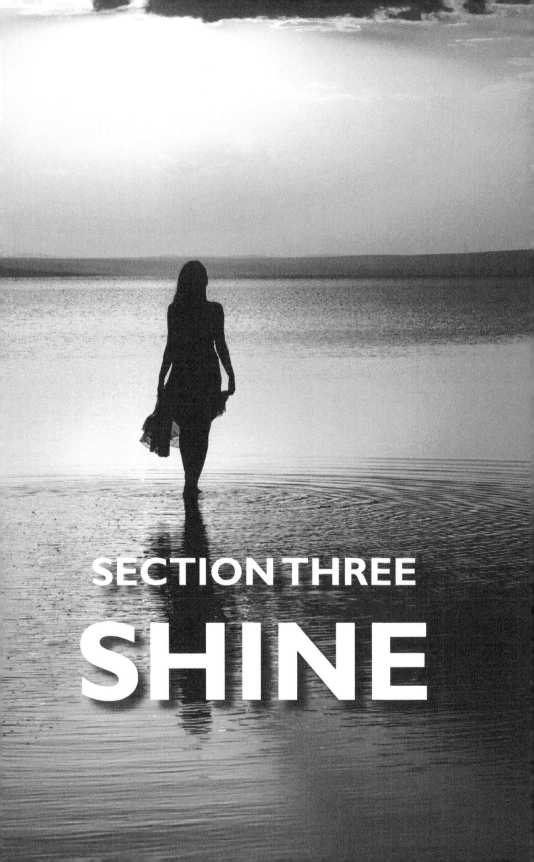

SECTION THREE

SHINE

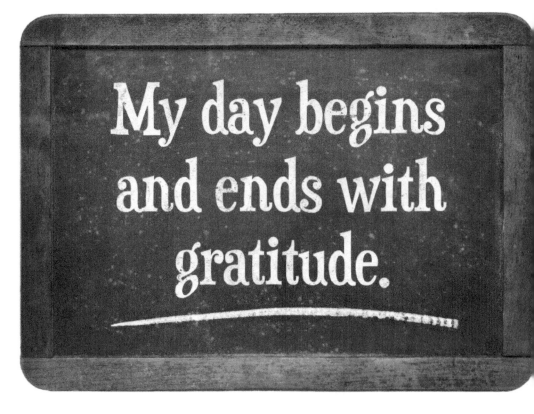

SECTION 3:
SHINE - Emotional Health

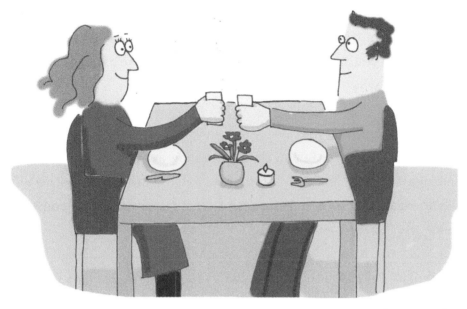

Being authentic, expressive and living my truth are all ideals I strive for. Why? Because I have learned that when I am authentic, expressive and living my truth, I am a happy person. I enjoy life much more, have more to give, and I am way more fun to be around. I like to call this journey "becoming myself, being free to be ME".

During my adult life, I have learnt just how important it is to keep growing and developing self-awareness. I find it liberating to tell the truth to myself about a situation and how I feel, without judging myself. Life becomes better, there is more fun, more love and laughter.

I have been enjoying the practice of 'taking in the good', which is explained by Rick Hanson in his book *Hardwiring Happiness*. He explains that as a survival strategy thousands of years ago, our brains evolved so that we held onto bad experiences like Velcro holds on, yet let go of good ones as if they were sliding off Teflon.

This new practice is rather like re-wiring the brain and only takes about a dozen seconds, a few times a day, to actually make changes. How you do this is by dwelling for slightly longer than normal (about 10 to 12 seconds) on a good experience, e.g. watching your dog play, or the pleasure of a cup of coffee, or the satisfaction of doing a job you had been avoiding. By dwelling on it, you are giving yourself a prolonged sense of peace, love and contentment, which become habitual qualities.

We all know only too well that stress makes us unhappy and massively contributes to disease. But stress is not going away any time soon. The challenge is how to handle the internal and external stresses of life, develop skills to deal with these stresses, and create appropriate responses to them.

Psychologist Kelly McGonigal, in a 2013 TED talk, (Ref. 1) urges us to see stress as a positive. She also reveals in her book (Ref. 2) that how you think about stress matters. Rather than get rid of stress, she says you need to change your view of stress. Stress is your body helping you to rise to the challenge.

1 She suggests that if you see your pounding heart as no problem, that it is helping you deal better with the situation, this gives you strength and energy to deal with the situation. If you view breathing faster as fine, appreciating that it is getting more oxygen to your brain, then it has been shown your blood vessels actually stay relaxed as happens in moments of joy and courage, rather than constricting as in a heart attack. So choosing to view your stress response to be helpful, you create a biology of courage and resilience.

2 Stress makes you social and motivates you to give and seek support through the action of oxytocin, normally known as the cuddle hormone. Oxytocin acts in the body as a natural anti-inflammatory, keeping blood vessels relaxed. It also acts as a neurohormone in the brain priming you to do things that strengthen close relationships, enhancing empathy, and making you more willing to help and support people you care about.

She concludes that it's best to go after that which creates meaning in your life and trust yourself to be able to handle the stress that follows.

I recently read about a wise 92-year-old lady, whom we can learn from. She says:

"Happiness is something you decide on ahead of time. Whether I like my room or not doesn't depend on how the furniture is arranged, it's how I arrange my mind. I already decided to love it. It's a decision I make every morning when I wake up."

She adds, "Remember the five simple rules to be happy:

1. Free your heart from hatred
2. Free your mind from worries
3. Live simply
4. Give more
5. Expect less

Ten Ways to Shine

Here are 10 ways to increase the experience of happiness and emotional well-being, that have helped me and countless others.

1. Choose Gratitude

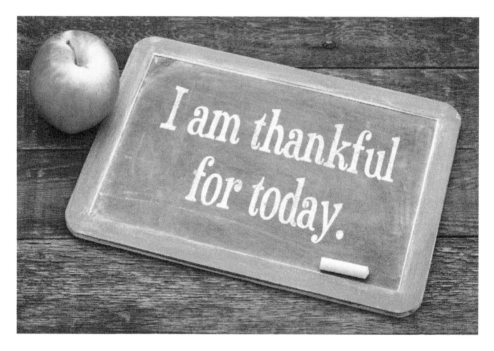

I sometimes consider my mind to be rather like a machine, chattering away churning out one negative disempowering thought after another. When I bring my awareness to this, I am more able to interrupt the flow; then I bring a small smile to my face, feeling instantly better, and thank myself for this break from my mind. I start to describe what I am grateful for in this moment: my breath, a stretch, a yawn bringing my awareness of sensation into the experience, creating a somatic moment. Then I go on to include gratitude for my family, my health, and on and on.

Starting each day with gratitude has become an amazing practice, ever since hearing Louise Hay describe how she thanks her mattress every morning for the night's sleep. Somehow my brain is 'tricked' into being positive even when the natural drift, first thing in the morning, is less than positive. And I consider myself to be a pretty optimistic person.

An article published in the *Harvard Mental Health Newsletter* stated, "Expressing thanks may be one of the simplest ways to feel better." (Ref. 1) Studies have shown that gratitude can produce measurable changes in the stress hormone cortisol, plus an increase in the pleasure-related neurotransmitter dopamine, oxytocin and seratonin. (Ref. 2)

Sometimes I keep a gratitude journal, writing down three good things that happened to me during that day. Another way is to keep a gratitude jar. This jar contains small pieces of paper that members of the family write on and place in the jar. Writing what you are grateful for can be spontaneous, at any time, then folded and placed in the jar. Once a week, maybe during a meal or at any other time, some of the papers can be withdrawn and read. It's a lovely time to appreciate each other too.

2. Emotional Freedom Technique (EFT)
also called Tapping

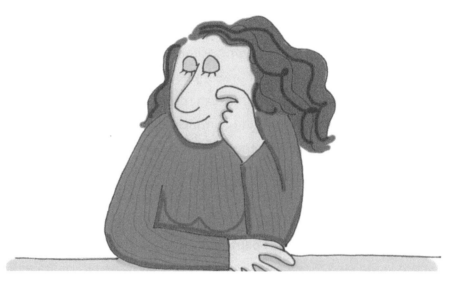

This is one of my favourite techniques for reducing anxiety and has made a huge difference to my sense of peace and equanimity. Taking a couple of courses in EFT with Peter and Tamara Donn, EFT Master Trainers, has enabled me to feel that I have this method available at my fingertips!

Here's what Peter says about EFT:

"Emotional Freedom Techniques (EFT) has been rapidly growing in popularity over the past two decades. It is like acupuncture for the emotions (but uses no needles) and is getting its reputation from its ability to improve your emotional state commonly within seconds or minutes, and often dramatically.

It can be used in two ways:

1. to lift and release current negative emotions
2. to amplify a positive feeling you want to feel

Although you can see professionally trained EFT practitioners to receive help in any area of life, it is simple enough to use on your own for self-help in countless ways, and on a daily basis, if needed.

EFT involves tapping lightly on a small set of acupuncture points whilst focusing on what you'd like to work on and stating a word or phrase describing the related feelings. What happens is quite remarkable. If you are focusing on general stress, for example, you find it starts to dissolve. If you are focusing on an upsetting feeling triggered by a hurtful comment (for example, a feeling of anger), this emotion starts to release, revealing a deeper layer (for example, feeling misunderstood in this case). By releasing each successive layer, a deep state of well-being and peace is reached.

This same process can be used for fear of something happening in the future, or general anxiety, or a feeling of overwhelm. It is particularly powerful when used on past upsetting experiences and traumas. In many cases, complete relief can be obtained within a 15 to 60 minutes period to the point where you can't get upset, even if you tried! You feel clear, light and peaceful, and often spontaneous forgiveness is experienced. This allows the past to no longer have any hold over you, and so it is easier to live in the stillness of the present moment where true joy and happiness resides.

EFT can also be used to elevate a positive state of being you would like to experience called "Positive EFT". You can be wildly imaginative with this. For example, you can state: "I want to feel completely carefree in my life," and as you move around the tapping points, you experience that particular experience becoming stronger and stronger.

Other examples may be:

"I want to have more joy in my life"

"The energy of golden sunlight"

"Sea breeze"

"A deep sense of safety and being taken care of"

"I want to feel Ghandi's presence and wisdom within me"

You can learn the basics for free, from manuals and YouTube videos. However, good training will give you the skills to understand how to apply EFT properly and learn how to get deep change. There are different training organisations such as the AAMET (www.aamet.org), The AMT (www.theamt.com) or EFT Universe (www.eftuniverse.com).

I can recommend Peter's courses listed on his website www.eft-courses.org.uk where he also offers a free online manual, which can get you started straight away.

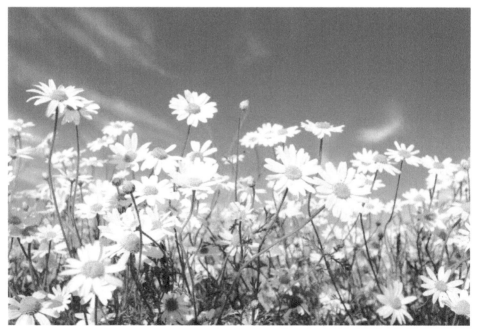

3. Nature

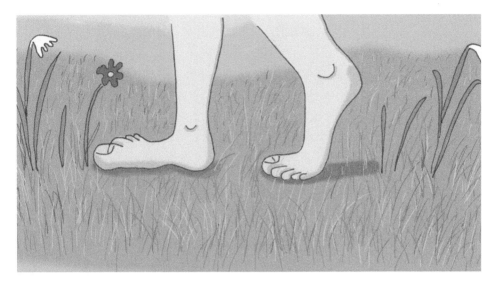

Nature is a wonderful healer. Get outside, find some nature, even in a city park. Whatever the weather, enjoy all the seasons. I have to admit that as I get older, spring has become my favourite season. But whatever the month, I take great pleasure in looking at, listening to, and inhaling all that is around me as I spend time in woods, walking across fields, along footpaths ... oh, the joys of having a dog to walk. He makes me get out there at least twice a day!

In the warm months, I love to sit on the grass in the garden and walk around barefoot to benefit from connecting to the earth – called grounding or earthing. This enables electrons from the Earth to flow through the bare feet and into the body. These electrons neutralise free radicals, reducing inflammation and aging. Stephen Sinatra, author of *Earthing*, discusses research that has demonstrated it takes about 80 minutes for the free electrons from the earth to fully reach your bloodstream and transform your blood, but any amount of time is beneficial. (Ref. 1)

4. Mindfulness – becoming aware

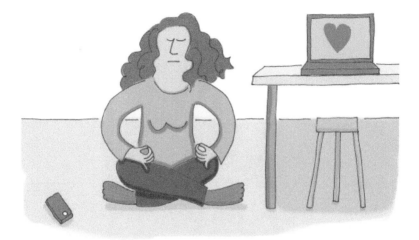

Quite a buzz word these days, 'mindfulness' is often used synonymously with 'meditation'. Far from the purpose of mindfulness being about changing and improving yourself or immunising yourself against any bad feelings, ever again, it is about being with things just the way they are, about knowing yourself and being yourself, even more.

For many years, I held the view that I 'should' meditate, that it would be good for me, give me more of a sense of peace and help me de-stress; I just didn't quite make the time for it, not even five minutes a day. Recently, my daughter and her partner were staying with us for a month, and at some point, they wildly suggested we get together at 6.30 a.m. to meditate for an hour! What a way to start the day! To my great surprise, I took to it, and continued the practice on my own after they left.

The practice of meditating for a fixed amount of time, be it five to ten minutes, or even an hour, is known as formal mindfulness or meditation. It usually involves sitting, but can be done standing, walking or even lying down. During this quiet time, I learned to rest in the silence, allowing my thoughts to come and go and not be attached to any of them. I also learned to gently bring my attention back to the present without giving myself a hard time about wandering off in my thoughts. After all, that is the nature of the mind. I also like to recite to myself and ponder on a Meditation or Verse by Rudolf Steiner. (Ref. 1)

Another form of mindfulness is known as informal practice, which involves bringing awareness to everyday activities; becoming aware and present while waiting for the kettle to boil, sitting in traffic, walking the dog etc. As I continue to practice daily, I notice more room for self-compassion and a sense of calmness. This awareness reminds me that my life is about so much more than what is on my to-do list for the day. I also recommend practicing mindful eating so that you can actually feel what foods work for you (see Chapter 1.) You are your own best healer.

In the film *Kung Fu Panda*, the quote from the wise Grand Master Oogway is a favourite of mine:

"You are too concerned about what was and what will be. There is a saying: yesterday is history, tomorrow is a mystery, but today is a gift. That is why it is call the 'Present'."

Jon Kabat Zin, teacher and author renowned for his books on mindfulness, in a recent interview (Mindfulness Summit 2015) shared that he sees meditation as a 'radical act of love and sanity'.

And I like how he invited the meditator to rest, "in the silence in between and underneath my words, a silence that is never not here, never broken, infinitely and always available to you.

"Not only to befriend but to inhabit moment by moment, by timeless moment, as we sit here with life unfolding exactly the way life is unfolding in this moment, so we don't have to achieve any particular feeling or state, or pursue anything but put the welcome mat out for whatever is here, including the unwanted, the unpleasant, the full catastrophe, so to speak and rest in awareness, fully embodied and fully awake."

Energy Boosting Tip
from Joanna Hill, Director of The Bagnall Centre
for Integrated Health
www.bagnallcentre.com

"Take the time to stop, turn off your phone and iPod, breathe, and savour a beautiful scene, such as an amazing sunset, a lovely animal, or a stunning tree in its autumn colours. If only for a minute, it will cost nothing, and make you smile for the rest of the day."

As mindfulness becomes more mainstream, it is being discussed and even practiced in the Houses of Commons and Lords in the British Parliament, as well as in some primary schools and businesses. Mindfulness Based Stress Reduction (MBSR) courses are available as a way to reduce stress and live life more fully. There is no promise that your stress will go away, but more that you can change your relationship to stress and everything else in your life; as you exercise that muscle of mindfulness, so everything in your life becomes your practice, your whole life, and not just how long you sit in the morning or evening.

I love this illustration of mindfulness:

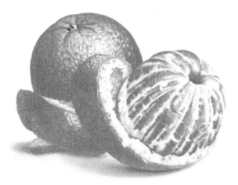

"Take the time to eat an orange in mindfulness. If you eat an orange in forgetfulness, caught in your anxiety and sorrow, the orange is not really there. But if you bring your mind and body together to produce true presence, you can see that the orange is a miracle. Peel the orange. Smell the fruit. See the orange blossoms in the orange, and the rain and the sun that have gone through the orange blossoms. The orange tree that has taken several months to bring this wonder to you. Put a section in your mouth, close your mouth mindfully, and with mindfulness feel the juice coming out of the orange."

Thich Nhat Hanh
The Moment is Perfect, Shambhala Sun, May 2008.

5. Flow writing

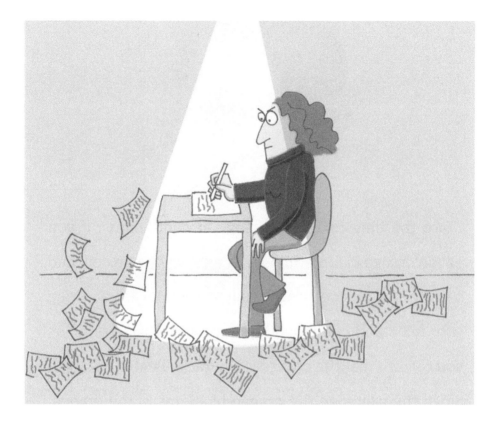

Do you ever feel like you have to censor what you want to say, so that you are acceptable and appear to be understanding of someone else? When inside there is another conversation going on that would be too risky to reveal? After all, we generally would like to avoid being blunt and hurtful to others. Of course, there is a time and place to talk straight, but it is not always appropriate to give your full and valid opinion. So flow writing is a way to let the thoughts be liberated, not bottled up with emotions. It stops them from festering and causing dis-ease.

Flow writing starts with just letting the pen travel across the page as the words flow, also called stream of consciousness. Julia Cameron, in *The Artist's Way*, calls this exercise 'Morning Pages', and she suggests writing three sides of A4 every morning. You don't need to feel good at writing, nor watch your grammar or spellings, because no one is going to judge you, or even read it. No planning is needed, just say on paper how it is right now; even, "I just don't know what to write" or, "Now my hand is aching from all this writing". And knowing that at the end it is fine to either keep the paper, throw it away or even burn it, is freeing. Plus it is a wonderful way to get to know yourself!

Dr David Hanscom, an orthopedic surgeon in Seattle, encourages patients with chronic back pain to practice expressive writing, where you write down your negative thoughts. It breaks up the psychological pathways of anxiety and frustration, allowing you to reprogram your brain and release physical pain. He describes success stories in his book *Back in Control: A spine surgeon's roadmap out of chronic pain*.

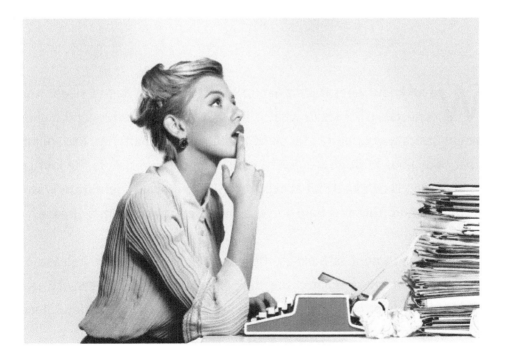

6. Sleeping well

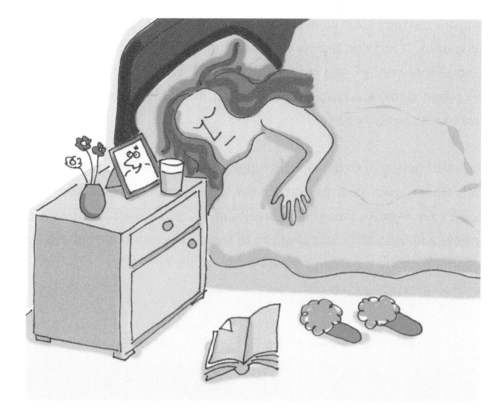

We all know what if feels like to have had a bad night's sleep. And conversely, we know what it feels like to have had a good night's sleep! Basically your body uses sleep to recharge the batteries. Each night, your body goes through a detoxification process. An article in the journal *Science* (Ref. 1) revealed that at night there is a removal of neurotoxic waste from the brain. This may help prevent the onset of Alzheimer's disease.

A dark environment is best as this allows for an optimum release of melatonin, which stimulates the deep healing sleep we need, so use blackout blinds or curtains if you have lights outside your window. Sleep masks work for some.

Energy Boosting Tip

from Dora Roszik-Csendes, Complementary Therapist

www.thelovingpresenceproject.com

"SLEEEEEEP!!!! Go to bed early (before 10 p.m.), or if you haven't had enough or good enough sleep at night, try to squeeze in an afternoon nap. It's magic!

Not only do I feel more energised when I'm rested, but also more patient and kinder with others, more creative, more sociable, funnier and lighter."

7. Play

Dance, sing, tell stories and listen to the silence

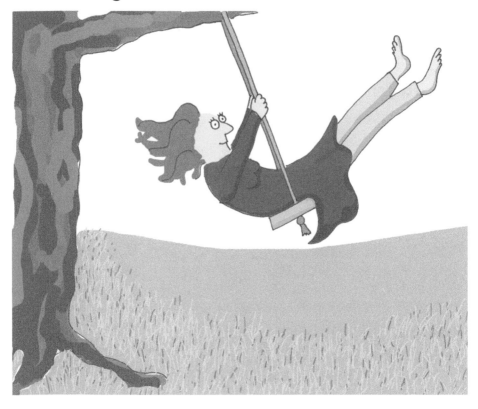

Play! Humour, laughter and joy are so healing for body and soul.

In many shamanic societies, if you came to a shaman or medicine person complaining of being disheartened, dispirited, or depressed, they would ask one of four questions.

- When did you stop dancing?
- When did you stop singing?
- When did you stop being enchanted by stories?
- When did you stop finding comfort in the sweet territory of silence?

Where we have stopped dancing, singing, being enchanted by stories, or finding comfort in silence, is where we have experienced the loss of soul.

"Dancing, singing, storytelling, and silence are the four universal healing salves."

Gabrielle Roth

I love all four of these questions, but the first one links directly with my passion for Nia movement. A student spontaneously said at the end of one of my Nia classes, "Nia is Joy without the drugs". She went on to expand that with Nia, young people would have no need to take the drug ecstasy.

Health Boosting Tip
from Danyah Miller, Storyteller
www.danyahmillerstoryteller.co.uk

"Stories are health-giving and life-affirming. When someone truly listens to another, it is deeply nourishing and healing. Stories make us laugh and cry, take us to places we may never otherwise know, we see ourselves reflected in them, empathise with others, and make connections that ordinarily pass us by. Telling stories is a way to share our collective history and our personal experiences, is a part of what makes us human. A wise person once remarked to me (quoting philosopher, Epictetus) that we have two ears and one mouth, and that we would do well if we used them in that ratio."

8. Relax by knitting

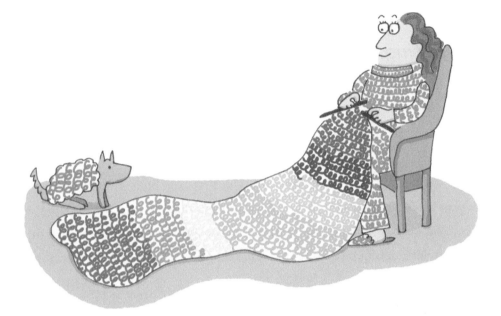

I know this does not appeal to everyone, but I have been knitting from the age of about seven, and although there have been times, even years, when I did not knit, I would predict that I have had some kind of knitting project on the go for about three quarters of my life. I find it an exciting and fulfilling way to express my creativity using my hands, as my patchwork blanket illustrates! And I love choosing colours, textures of yarn and patterns. Sharing this enthusiasm for yarns and patterns with dear knitting friends is part of the experience.

Knitting has been shown to release dopamine, a feel-good neurotransmitter. In a study of 3,500 knitters, by *The British Journal of Occupational Therapy*, 81% of respondents with depression said they felt happy after knitting — more than half took it even further and said they felt "very happy". (Ref. 1)

It has also been shown that knitting (and other crafts) help fight off dementia. When hands are used for these crafts in middle age, then cognitive impairment and memory loss in later years decreased by 30 to 50% (Ref 2.)

In Steiner (Waldorf) Education, all children learn to knit around the age of six to seven years old, and there is a saying, "nimble fingers, nimble mind". It's been scientifically proven that using your hands in a productive way triggers activity in 60% of your brain, which in later life can reduce the odds of dementia. It's also a wonderful way to stay calm and it has been shown that the repetitive actions of knitting activate the calming parasympathetic nervous system. Other crafts like patchwork would do this too.

Finally, you burn an amazing 55 kcal per hour while you knit, which is nicely balanced by two squares of dark chocolate containing about 50 kcal. Knitting offset!

9. Read Inspirational poems

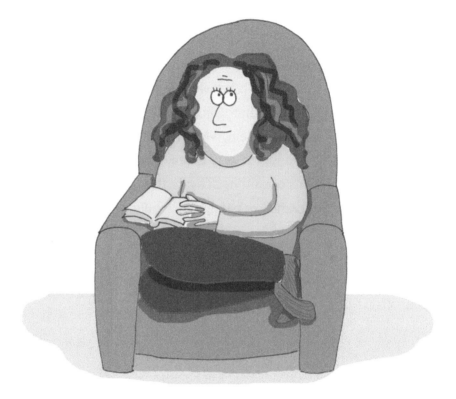

I no longer want to be Better than you

In my heart of hearts,
I no longer want to be
Better than you
Smarter than you
Thinner than you
Prettier than you
Faster than you
Stronger than you
More accomplished than you
More creative than you

A better mother than you
A better friend than you
Better educated than you
ANYTHING more than you.

I want to walk this path
Side by side
In awe of who you are
In awe of what your gifts are
To see you only in love and light
With your beauty shining through
Just as you are.
And I want you to see me the same way.
For I really do love you
Just as you are.
I only thought I had to be better
In order for you to love me.

I drop this cloak of outshining at the gate.
It has been such a heavy burden,
An unnecessary burden
A self imposed burden.
Will you still love me
Being just as I am.
In my heart of hearts,
I know you will.

Katy Stevenson Wirth

10. Ways to reduce stress and increase pleasure

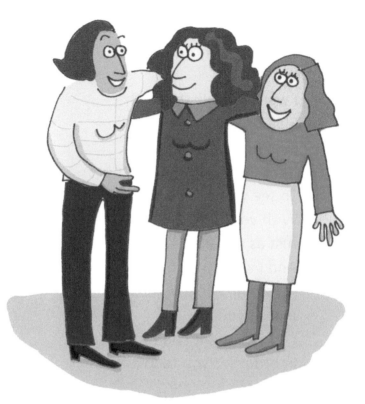

Energy Boosting Tip
from Dawn Golten

- Cook a fabulous meal for my friends and/or family, and include the most vital and alive food I can find.
- Leave my diary and work at home, and spend the day with my loved ones doing not very much.
- Do a complicated task that I have been putting off for a long time. Take a risk in my work, and push my knowledge and experience into new frontiers.
- Keep the commitment I have made to myself to grow a part of myself every day.

Most of us have heard of natural opiates in the brain called endorphins that makes us feel happy. There are some easy ways to increase the amount circulating:

get connected

with friends and family and have a good chat, catch up, crack jokes, and remember that gossip does not have to have a negative tone. We are social creatures and gossiping stimulates pleasure centres in the brain and releases endorphins. Have a chat with a good friend; being heard is sometimes all that is needed, not loads of advice or opinions. Other times, what is needed is a professional counsellor or psychotherapist.

laughter

you may well know that laughter makes you happy. Obviously! So look out for a funny film, share a joke, or remember a funny situation. Belly laughter is the best, as it involves your whole body. You could even try Laughter Yoga. I once took a class and loved it!

Energy Boosting Tip
from Melanie Bloch, Holistic Laughter Coach
www.melaniebloch.co.uk

A great stress releasing and energising Laughter Yoga exercise which encourages mind body connection awareness is "Body Scan Laughter"

1. Bring soft awareness to your scalp -gently rub your scalp - what sound do you want to make?
2. Now focus on your forehead, gently rub it - what sound do you want to make?
3. Continue focusing on eyes, nose, cheeks, mouth, jaw, throat, shoulders, arms, chest, stomach, gut, hips, legs, feet, toes.

4. Don't judge the sounds. It can be any of the following: pain release groans, 'aaaha' laughter, nasal laughter, humming, yawning, coughing.

dark chocolate

(Ref. 1 and Chapter 13) Just one square is enough to lift your mood, eaten slowly.

smelling vanilla or lavender

has also been shown to stimulate endorphin release. (Ref. 2)

exercise, another reason to get moving!

be open to love,

romantic and platonic, as a great way to increase the happiness in your life. Pet animals can also be a wonderful way to receive and give love.

Our black wooly dog, Teddy, has been a great source of love in our family. And when humans cuddle, even a pet animal, the cuddle hormone, oxytocin, is released in the brain, which researchers are testing for relief from depression. (Ref. 3)

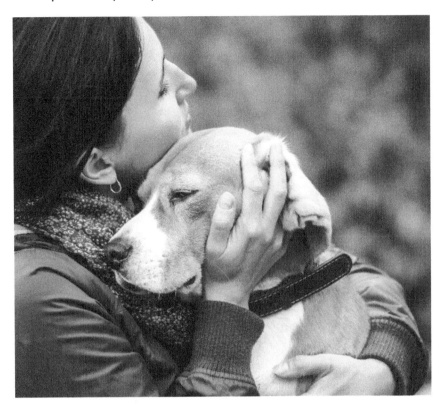

smiling

did you know, even a small smile can cause a relaxation of facial muscles and a release of endorphins and serotonin in your brain – the happy chemicals. Smiling also activates your zygomaticus major muscle, a muscle that is linked to your thymus gland, which is the 'school and factory' for your white blood cells, which are responsible for immune system strength.

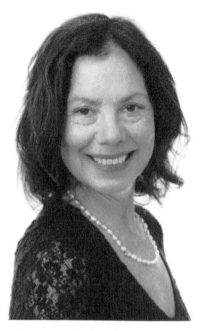

Here we are, at the end of this book. I hope you have enjoyed the ride. The ways to push back the years and feel amazing, discussed in *Eat Dance Shine*, are on the one hand simple, yet not always easy. I acknowledge your commitment to well-being and longevity.

I hope that this is only the beginning for you:

- in becoming even more aware of what makes you feel well; the benefits of eating plants, gradually finding more ways to increase your intake of whole, organic, ripe vegetables and fruits, and at the same time reducing foods that do not support your body.

- finding exercise and movement that you love and can enjoy several times a week.

- exploring some of the ways to 'Shine', to increase the experience of happiness and emotional well-being, and to create new neural pathways to happiness.

I hope that you are making friends with your 'inner guru'? Are you more aware of what works, knowing that you are unique, connecting more with your inner world, trusting your intuition, and actually feeling what is right for you?

Only you know what it really feels like to live in your body. You really are your own best healer.

I'd really like to hear from you, with any stories or questions that arise. Let me know how you get on with creating new habits to stay healthy as you *Eat Dance Shine*. Please get in touch.

If you are interested in my Green Nutrition workshops and Nia classes, details are on my website as well as my blog for the latest new healthy tips and ideas.

Warm wishes,

Michele

www.michelekaye.com

07786 172407

michele@michelekaye.com

https://www.facebook.com/michele.kaye

Twitter @michelekaye

Resources

Food and supplements

- Vegetarian omega-3 capsules (Echiomega) http://shop.igennus.com/
- Linseeds and linseed oil www.thelinseedfarm.co.uk
- Biona Capers in olive oil
- Orgran no egg (gluten free)
- Ocean's Alive Marine Phytoplankton

Vitamin D3

- Better U Vitamin D spray
- Vitamin D3 capsules from Ancient Purity (http://www.ancientpurity.com/)
- Grassroots Health – Vitamin D Action, Carole Braggley, Director of Grassroots Health, a public Health Promotion Organization http://www.grassrootshealth.net/

Organic vegetables and fruit suppliers:

- Abel & Cole
- Riverford

Inspiration for growing edible plants:

- 'Incredible Edible' http://www.incredible-edible-todmorden.co.uk/
- 'Guerrilla Gardening' http://www.guerrillagardening.org/

Chocolate:

- Lovechock
- Conscious Chocolate
- Raw Chocolate Company
- Raw cocoa nibs

Water bottle:

- i9 Informed Water Bottle   http://i9bottle.com/

Cleaning products:

- Ecover
- Bio-D
- Libby Chan cleaning products

Books

- *The Artist's Way* by Julia Cameron (Pan, 1995)

- *Supplements Exposed* by Brian R. Clement (Career Press/New Page Books, 2009)

- *Mindful Eating* by Jan Chozen Bays (Shambhala Publications Inc, 2009)

- *The Yoga of Eating* by Charles Eisenstein (New Trends Publishing Inc, 2009)

- *Fats that Heal, Fats that Kill* by Udo Erasmus (Alive Books, 1993)

- *Healing the Gerson Way: Defeating Cancer and other Chronic Diseases* by Charlotte Gerson with Beata Bishop (Gerson Health Media, 2010)

- *Imperfectly Natural Woman* by Janey Lee Grace (Crown House Publishing, 2005)

- *Hardwiring Happiness* by Rick Hanson (Rider, 2014)

- *Earthing: The Most Important Health Discovery Ever?* by Clint Ober and Dr Sinatra (Basic Health Publications, Inc., 2014)

- *Food Rules: An Eater's Manual* by Michael Pollan (Penguin, 2010)

- *The Nia Technique: The High-Powered Energizing Workout That Gives You a New Body and a New Life* by Carlos Rosas, Debbie Rosas (Harmony, 2005)

- *Vegetable Juicing for Everyone* by Dr Andrew Saul (Basic Health Publications, 2013)

- *Verses and Meditations* by Rudolf Steiner (Rudolf Steiner Press, 1972)

- *The Rainbow Diet* by Chris Woollams (Health Issues Ltd, 2015)

References

For website addresses of articles, see Reference page on
www.michelekaye.com

Section 1. EAT

Chapter 1. Dietary dogma versus Freedom

1. Jan Chozen Bays, *Mindful Eating*

Chapter 2. Love plants

1. George TW1, Waroonphan S, Niwat C, Gordon MH, Lovegrove JA. *Effects of acute consumption of a fruit and vegetable purée-based drink on vasodilation and oxidative status.* British Journal of Nutrition. 2013 Apr 28;109(8):1442-52.

2.Philip J Tuso, MD, Mohamed H Ismail, MD, [...], and Carole Bartolotto, MA, RD *Nutritional Update for Physicians: Plant-Based Diets*

3. Pallauf K, Rimbach G. *Autophagy, polyphenols and healthy ageing.* Ageing Res Rev 2012, 12(1):237-252. PubMed Abstract

4. Salminen A, Kaarniranta K, Kauppinen A: *Inflammaging: disturbed interplay between autophagy and inflammasomes.* Aging (Albany NY) 2012, 4(3):166-175.

Chapter 3. Eat a rainbow

1. Bishayee A1, Mbimba T, Thoppil RJ, Háznagy-Radnai E, Sipos P, Darvesh AS, Folkesson HG, Hohmann J. *Anthocyanin-rich black currant (Ribes*

nigrum L.) extract affords chemoprevention against diethylnitrosamine-induced hepatocellular carcinogenesis in rats. J Nutr Biochem. 2011 Nov;22(11):1035-46.

2. Leonardi M. *Treatment of fibrocystic disease of the breast with myrtillus anthocyanins. Our experience.* [Article in Italian] Minerva Ginecol. 1993 Dec;45(12):617-21.

3. Johnson SA, Figueroa A, Navaei N, Wong A, Kalfon R, Ormsbee LT, Feresin RG, Elam ML, Hooshmand S, Payton ME, Arjmandi BH. *Daily blueberry consumption improves blood pressure and arterial stiffness in postmenopausal women with pre- and stage 1-hypertension: a randomized, double-blind, placebo-controlled clinical trial.* J Acad Nutr Diet. 2015 Mar;115(3):369-77.

4. Adams LS1, Zhang Y, Seeram NP, Heber D, Chen S. *Pomegranate ellagitannin-derived compounds exhibit antiproliferative and antiaromatase activity in breast cancer cells in vitro.* Cancer Prev Res (Phila). 2010 Jan;3(1):108-13

5. The Age-Related Eye Disease Study 2 (AREDS2) Research Group. *Lutein + Zeaxanthin and Omega-3 Fatty Acids for Age-Related Macular Degeneration* The Age-Related Eye Disease Study 2 (AREDS2) Randomized Clinical Trial

6. Healwithfood.org/health-benefits/sweet-potatoes-purple-orange

7. Webmed.com/vitamins-supplements/ingredientmono-554-lycopene.

8. Duo J1, Ying GG, Wang GW, Zhang L. *Quercetin inhibits human breast cancer cell proliferation and induces apoptosis via Bcl-2 and Bax regulation.* Mol Med Rep. 2012 Jun;5(6):1453-6.

9. Aherne SA1, O'Brien NM. *Dietary flavonols: chemistry, food content, and metabolism.* Nutrition. 2002 Jan;18(1):75-81.

Chapter 4. Grapes and Wine

1. Patient.co.uk/health/alcohol-and-sensible-drinking

2. Huffingtonpost.com/dr-mercola/if-you-want-to-age-gracefully

Chapter 5. The ultimate fast food - JUICES

1. Garnett Cheney *Rapid healing of peptic ulcers in patients receiving fresh cabbage juice* Calif Med. Jan 1949; 70(1): 10–15.

2. Ayman I Elkady, Osama A Abuzinadah, Nabih A Baeshen, Tarek R Rahmy. Differential Control of Growth, *Apoptotic Activity, and Gene Expression in Human Breast Cancer Cells by Extracts Derived from Medicinal Herbs Zingiber officinale.* J Biomed Biotechnol. 2012 ;2012:614356.

3. Mercola.com/2014/06/26/supporting evidence for Aspartame-Alzheimer's Link Emerges

Chapter 7. Fatty Fishy Facts

1. PhysiciansCommittee for Responsible Medicine.org/health/health-topics/essential-fatty-acids

2. Webmd.com/diet/features/what-to-know-about-omega-3s-and-fish

3. TAB Sanders, MC Hochland *A comparison of the influence on plasma lipids and platelet function of supplements of ω3 and ω6 polyunsaturated fatty acids* British Journal of Nutrition (1 983), 50, 521-529

4. Udo Erasmus *Fats that Heal Fats that Kill*

5. Cristina Augood, Usha Chakravarthy, Ian Young, Jesus Vioque, Paulus TVM de Jong, Graham Bentham, Mati Rahu, Johan Seland, Gisele Soubrane, Laura Tomazzoli, Fotis Topouzis, Johannes R Vingerling, and Astrid E Fletcher *Oily fish consumption, dietary docosahexaenoic acid and eicosapentaenoic acid intakes, and associations with neovascular age-related macular degeneration1,2,3* Am J Clin Nutr August 2008 vol. 88 no. 2 398-406

6. Clement, B *Supplements Exposed 2010*

7. Maki KC, Rains TM *Stearidonic acid raises red blood cell membrane eicosapentaenoic acid.* J Nutr. 2012 Mar;142(3

8. Culinate.com/articles/culinate8/small_fish_mackerel

9. David Wolfe.com/fukushima-radiation-tumors-fish-seafood

10. Ikonomou, M.G., Higgs, D.A. et al. Department of Fisheries and Oceans (DFO), Institute of Ocean Sciences, British Columbia, Canada. *Flesh quality of market-size farmed and wild British Columbia salmon.* Environmental Science and Technology, 2007 Jan 15; 41(2): 437-43.

11. Kelly, B.C., Ikonomou, M.G. et al. Fisheries and Oceans Canada, Institute of Ocean Sciences, British Columbia, Canada. *Flesh residue concentrations of organochlorine pesticides in farmed and wild salmon from British Columbia, Canada.* Environmental Toxicology and Chemistry, 2011 Nov; 30(11): 2456-64.

12. Mozaffarian, D., Rimm E.B. *Fish intake, contaminants, and human health: evaluating the risks and the benefits.* Journal of the American Medical Association, 2006 Oct 18; 296(15):1885-99.

13. Greatist.com/health/farmed-wild-salmon-health-environment

14.Healthimpactnews.com/2014/mct-oil-vs-coconut-oil-the-truth-exposed

Chapter 10. Supplements

1. Clement B. *Supplements Exposed 2010*

2. Prof Isobel Jennings *Vitamins in Endocrine Metabolism*

Chapter 11. Vitamin D and Cancer prevention

1. Fresh-network.blog/2010/02/are-you-getting-enough-vitamin-d

2. International Agency for Research on Cancer. *GLOBOCAN 2012: estimated cancer incidence, mortality and prevalence worldwide in 2012.* Lyon, France: International Agency for Research on Cancer/World Health Organization; 2012. Pages/fact_sheets_cancer.

3. Sharif B. Mohr, Edward D. Gorham, June Kim, Heather Hofflich and Cedric F. Garland. *Meta-analysis of Vitamin D Sufficiency for Improving Survival of Patients with Breast Cancer* ANTICANCER RESEARCH 34: 1163-1166 (2014)

4. Lappe JM1, Travers-Gustafson D, Davies KM, Recker RR, Heaney RP. *Vitamin D and calcium supplementation reduces cancer risk: results of a randomized trial* Am J Clin Nutr June 2007

5. Vitamindcouncil.org/blog/dr-cannell-on-vitamin-k2

6. Mercola.com 2013/10/19/vitamin-d-vitamin-k2

Chapter 12. Superfoods

1. Mercola.com 2014/10/13/turmeric-curcumin.

2. IFT.org January 11, 2011 *curcumin-may-relieve-pain-inflammation-for-osteoarthritis-patients*

3. Greenmedinfo blog *600-reasons-turmeric-may-be-worlds-most-important-herb*

4. Oregon State University 2012/may/*curry-new-biological-role-identified-compound-used-ancient-medicine*

5. Mercola 2014/10/13/*turmeric-curcumin boosts regeneration of brain stem cells, and more*

Chapter 13. Chocolate revealed!

1. Scientific American article/*why-is-dark-chocolate-good-for-you-thank-your-microbes/*

Chapter 14. Clean Living

1.Human Exposome Project http://humanexposomeproject.com/

2. Oates, L, Cohen, M, Braun, L, Schembri, A and Taskova, R 2014, *'Reduction in urinary organophosphate pesticide metabolites in adults after a week-long organic diet'* Environmental Research, vol. 132, pp. 105-111.

Chapter 15. Making changes - one mouthful at a time

1. Prochaska and Diclemente 1982 *The Cycle of Change*

Section 2. DANCE

1. huffingtonpost.com/2013/06/24/*exercise-brown-fat-good-bad*

2. Ulf Ekelund, Heather A Ward, Teresa Norat, Jian'an Luan, Anne M May, Elisabete Weiderpass, Stephen S Sharp, Kim Overvad, Jane Nautrup Østergaard, Anne Tjønneland, Nina Føns Johnsen, Sylvie Mesrine, Agnes Fournier, Guy Fagherazzi, Antonia Trichopoulou, Pagona Lagiou, Dimitrios Trichopoulos, Kuanrong Li, Rudolf Kaaks, Pietro Ferrari, Idlir Licaj, Mazda Jenab, Manuela Bergmann, Heiner Boeing, Domenico Palli, Sabina Sieri, Salvatore Panico, Rosario Tumino, Paolo Vineis, Petra H Peeters, Evelyn Monnikhof, H Bas Bueno-de-Mesquita, J Ramon Quir os, Antonio Agudo, María-Jose S anchez, Jos e Mar ía Huerta, Eva Ardanaz, Larraitz Arriola, Bo Hedblad, Elisabet Wirfalt, Malin Sund, Mattias Johansson, Timothy J Key, Ruth C Travis, Kay-Tee Khaw, Søren Brage, Nicholas J Wareham, and Elio Riboli *Physical activity and all-cause mortality across levels of overall and abdominal adiposity in European men and women: the European Prospective Investigation into Cancer and Nutrition* Study AmJClinNut. First published ahead of print January 14, 2015

3. Graham A. Colditz MD, DrPH1,* and Kari Bohlke ScD2 *Priorities for the primary prevention of breast cancer* CA: A Cancer Journal for Clinicians Volume 64, Issue 3, pages 186–194, May/June 2014

4. Mandrola J *Seeing Exercise as the Best Medicine* . . .. Medscape. Oct 22, 2014.

5. Arbab-Zadeh A, Perhonen M, Howden E, et al. *Cardiac remodeling in response to 1 year of intensive endurance training.* Circulation 2014; DOI:10.1161/CIRCULATIONAHA.114.010775.

6. *what-educators-and-parents-should-know-about-neuroplasticity-learning-and-dance* Sharpbrains.com

7. Carlos Rosas, Debbie Rosas *The Nia Technique: The High-Powered Energizing Workout That Gives You a New Body and a New Life* Jan 2005

Section 3. SHINE - Emotional Health

1. TED talk with pyschologist Kelly McGonigal 2013

2. Kelly McGonigal *The Upside of Stress*

Chapter 1. Choosing gratitude
1. Harvard mental health letter 2011/November: in-praise-of-gratitude

2. ABC News Health science-Thankfulness

Chapter 2. Emotional Freedom Technique (EFT) also called Tapping

AAMET www.aamet.org
The AMT www.theamt.com
EFT Universe www.eftuniverse.com

Chapter 3. Nature
 1. Clint Ober and Dr. Sinatra 2010 *Earthing: The Most Important Health Discovery Ever?*

Chapter 4. Mindfulness – becoming aware

1. Rudolf Steiner *Verses and Meditations*

Chapter 6. Sleeping well

1. Mercola: *Lack of sleep may cause brain shrinkage* 2014/09/18

Chapter 8.   Relax by knitting

1. Riley, Jill; Corkhill, Betsan; Morris, Clare *The benefits of knitting for personal and social wellbeing in adulthood: findings from an international survey* The British Journal of Occupational Therapy, Volume 76, Number 2, February 2013, pp. 50-57(8)

2. Geda YE1, Topazian HM, Roberts LA, Roberts RO, Knopman DS, Pankratz VS, Christianson TJ, Boeve BF, Tangalos EG, Ivnik RJ, Petersen RC.*Engaging in cognitive activities, aging, and mild cognitive impairment: a population-based study.*2011 study from the Journal of Neuropsychiatry & Clinical Neurosciences

Chapter 10.   Ways to reduce stress and increase pleasure

1. Linda Ciampa *Researchers say chocolate triggers feel-good chemicals* CNN Febuary 14, 1996

2. Reader's Digest: *8-ways-to-naturally-increase-endorphins*

3. SIOBHAN O'CONNOR *Can Cuddling Cure Depression?* Prevention.com/ mind-body/emotional-health/oxytocin-help-depression FEBRUARY 29, 2012

Lightning Source UK Ltd.
Milton Keynes UK
UKOW07f0038110516

274013UK00011B/50/P